HOW TO USE HOMOEOPATHY

HOW TO USE HOMOEOPATHY

A Comprehensive Instruction Book

DR CHRISTOPHER HAMMOND MB BS LCH

With a foreword by
RT HON THE LORD COLWYN CBE BDS LDS RCS

ELEMENT

Shaftesbury, Dorset • Rockport, Massachusetts
Brisbane, Queensland

© Christopher Hammond 1991

First published by
Caritas Healthcare
in 1988

Revised edition published in Great Britain in 1991 by
Element Books Limited
Shaftesbury, Dorset SP7 8BP

Published in the USA in 1991 by
Element Books, Inc.
PO Box 830, Rockport, MA 01966

Published in Australia in 1992 by
Element Books Limited for
Jacaranda Wiley Limited
33 Park Road, Milton, Brisbane 4064

Reprinted April and September 1992
Reprinted May 1993
Reprinted May and October 1994
Reprinted 1995

Cover illustration by Miranda Gray
Cover design by Max Fairbrother
Designed by Pete Russell, Holdsworth Associates, Reading
Typeset by Footnote Graphics, Warminster, Wiltshire
Printed and bound in Great Britain by
J W Arrowsmith Limited, Bristol, Avon

British Library Cataloguing in Publication Data
Hammond Christopher, 1955–
How to use homoeopathy.-Rev.ed.
I. Title
615.532

Library of Congress Cataloging in Publication
Data available

ISBN 1–85230–208–9

Foreword

Ever since the beginning of the NHS, there have been many varied reviews with the common theme that modern western medicine is in crisis.

Hardly a day goes by without some reference to the subject in the newspapers, on radio or television. Despite the high levels of spending on the NHS, our standard of health has not improved substantially, demand for services has increased and the system has evolved as a sickness service, with very little to do with health.

Given the unhealthy lifestyles of most people and the extent to which we constantly abuse our bodies with social and clinical drugs, unsuitable diets and other varied stresses associated with our environment, it is not surprising that many people feel run down or even ill for much of the time. There are few signs that the NHS is doing anything to rectify the situation or even that it is capable of doing so.

Modern treatment therapy is quite helpless when faced with chronic diseases and is constantly reduced to providing merely palliative, rather than curative, treatment. The root cause of this inability to change can be found in the dominance of health-care services by Allopathic medicine, since it sets the tone for all official attitudes towards health.

The main aim of therapies which are designated alternative or complementary is to emphasise the basic importance of each individual doing as much as possible to maintain his or her own health, rather than being dependent on the GP or specialist.

Much more effort should be put into the promotion and enhancement of health, rather than waiting for people to become ill and then applying expensive medical techniques in disease management.

In this age of unprecedented technological advance, we also see unprecedented damage being done to the atmosphere, the water and the land. Human violations of the laws of nature result in the contamination of the environment and, in turn, place an increased stress on the ability of the individual to function. This, together with the fact that mankind has gradually lost the inner awareness which would have enabled the correct perception of, and respect for, the laws of nature means that we see, collectively and individually, human beings both affecting and being affected by the environment. As we deviate increasingly from the laws of nature, a vicious cycle is established which requires great insight and energy to correct.

For each individual in this situation there may be a wide variety of possible responses to external stresses. Some people seem to be relatively unaffected by external or internal disturbances. They are in a state of relative balance which is maintained with minimal effort. Most people, on the other hand, experience degrees of imbalance ranging from slight to very severe. These are the people we consider dis-eased in the broadest use of the term. In such people the disturbance manifests itself in a highly individualistic and varied manner, but always the disturbance can be viewed as an imbalance of the organism's ability to cope with external influences.

This is where the practice of Homoeopathy is such a useful bridge. Many of its practitioners have been through an orthodox medical education in disease management. Homoeopathic therapists are able to educate the public in the importance of a healthy lifestyle, explain the significance of our self-healing capacity and bring about the realisation that health care is much more about health promotion than about the alleviation of the symptoms of the disease.

Modern medical education is a poor basis for health promotion and the great range of problems in which mind, body and environment so obviously interact. The promotion of the Homoeopathic philosophy is of vital importance as we become aware of the increased significance of iatrogenic illness.

The first edition of this book received praise from the public and the Homoeopathic profession in this country and abroad. The second edition has several new sections and an improved layout. Dr Hammond successfully presents the benefits and philosophy of the Homoeopathic approach to health and the principles of an holistic view of treatment in the clearest terms. *How to Use Homoeopathy* provides both a practical and easy manual for first aid treatment and a workable model for patterns of health care for the future.

Rt. Hon. The Lord Colwyn CBE, BDS, LDS, RCS.

January 1991.

Acknowledgements

The list of people who have made a contribution to this book is enormous. Let me start by thanking my family who supported and encouraged me to write this book at the same time providing occasional opportunities to test the system in it when treating their ailments. In particular, I would like to thank my wife, Dr Jennifer Thomas who published the first edition under the label Caritas Healthcare, and Michael Mann of Element Books Ltd, for his willingness to distribute the home-spun first edition and for his enthusiasm in taking on the publication of this edition.

I wish to thank Robert Davidson for his excellent teaching of Homoeopathy and his inspiring vision for the future, Barbara Harwood for her energy and enthusiasm and Sheilagh Creasy for her experience and help with reading through the Tables and Materia Medica before publication of the first edition. I am indebted to Stephen Cummings and Dana Ullman for inspiration, particularly with the sections advising when to seek medical help. I owe gratitude to the many practitioners who have been kind enough to endorse and recommend the book to patients and students and encourage its expansion to include new material, particularly on women's ailments, in the second edition. David Howell has been especially helpful in this regard.

The great masters of the past need to be mentioned too, especially Dr Boericke whose system of analysing a case of illness inspired the layout of the tables designed to make this book easy to use, the classical Homoeopaths back to Hahnemann himself who reformulated the principles of Homoeopathy and earlier still Paracelsus, Aristotle, Charaka and many other great physicians for whom the principle of 'Like cures like' was a familiar basis for treatment.

Finally thanks are due to the patients who allow me to help them and in so doing teach me so much.

Contents

Appendix

PART 1

Homoeopathy:
The Theory and Practice

§1 The theory and philosophy of Homoeopathy

What is Homoeopathy?

Homoeopathy is a complete system of medicine which aims to promote general health, by reinforcing the body's own natural healing capacity. Homoeopathy does not have treatments for diseases. It has remedies for people with diseases.

It works in a totally different way from conventional medicine, which is known to Homoeopathic practitioners as Allopathy. Allopathy means 'different from the suffering'; the drugs that are given work against the disease and its symptoms. Therefore drugs that are 'anti' are found, such as anti-biotics, anti-depressants, anti-inflammatory and anti-pain drugs etc. Homoeopathy means 'similar to the suffering'. The remedies used to treat sick people are actually capable of producing similar symptoms and diseases to those present in the patient needing that remedy. The significance of this should become more clear to you as you read this chapter and you become familiar with the 'Homoeopathic' view of the world and its ills.

So how does Homoeopathy work? Before attempting to answer that question it is necessary to understand a little about the function of disease in our lives.

Does disease have a function?

It is often useful, when explaining a very large concept, to start at the beginning. In this case let us consider the healthy child and the illnesses that commonly occur in childhood. Healthy children have lots of energy as a rule, so much so that they can wear out their poor unhealthy parents! When they get ill, what sort of illnesses do they get? Do they not tend to get sick rapidly with a very high fever, a vigorous illness which puts them in bed? Then in a matter of days, or even one day, are they not up and about again eating us out of house and home? At least, is this not the tendency in the beginning with most very young children and certainly with lively, healthy ones?

So what is going on in illness? Sometimes an observant parent will notice something that will give us a clue; after a child recovers from one of those high fevers that 'lay it very low' for a short time it is sometimes seen that the child is more 'well' than before it became 'ill', provided the illness has not been inappropriately treated or interfered with in some way. Often this is very subtle. There may be an improvement in the child's already abundant energy or that nebulous sense of well being that we all know about but find so hard to put into words. This may show itself by an improvement in the child's behaviour or in the resolution of some lingering problem, such as the slight cough or persistently runny nose. Frequently this improvement is missed or does not occur because of some form of interference. If you have healthy young children, observe them closely and see what you can find out for yourself.

What happens as we grow up? There is a tendency for illnesses to become more prolonged, less intense and for the recovery to be slower. Eventually the recovery becomes incomplete and we can see the gradual emergence of chronic disease. From this progression it becomes possible to consider chronic diseases either as acute illnesses from which we have not been able to recover fully or as arising from the individual having insufficient 'energy', for whatever reason, to develop an acute illness and be done with it! Of course this can start in the very young, though it is much more rare.

Is chronic disease inevitable?

Why does this happen? What has gone wrong? Is it natural for man to slowly degenerate in this way? Just because it is so common that it is regarded as 'normal' to expect chronic ill health with advancing years does that mean that it is the way things have to be or, indeed, should be?

Occasionally we hear of people of very advanced years who appear and act as if they were in their prime, both mentally and physically. Plainly not everyone has to be subject to chronic disease. Is it not possible that these few exceptional individuals are, in fact, the normal ones and the rest of us have somewhere deviated from this path of health?

For me, it makes much more sense to look at the world from the point of view that things should be perfect. If they are not, something has interfered with the natural state and thrown things out of balance. This is of direct importance to the view of health and the function of disease in Homoeopathy.

Already we have looked at the healthy state of the majority of children when they enter this world and how their health tends to deteriorate slowly with time. This need not be considered 'normal' or inevitable.

When does disease begin?

This is the first point to consider. Let us look at an example of acute illness that would naturally resolve in time. We commonly think of an illness as starting when the symptoms commence, like the lethargy and runny nose at the beginning of a cold. To understand Homoeopathy we must consider a little more deeply and look at the situation afresh.

Consider a crowded bus in the rush hour. Right in the centre is one person with a streaming cold who is sneezing his head off! What happens next? During the following few days a number of people in the bus will go down with a cold and will likely blame the poor soul who was suffering on his journey home. But look a little more deeply and you will see that something else has happened too; if a number of people have gone down with the cold, does not it mean that a number of people have not gone down with the cold? So why, if the bugs that the sneezing man spread about the bus were the cause of the illness, did not everyone get a cold? What have we overlooked in blaming the man or his bugs for the cold?

It is, of course, quite obvious once we stop to think about it that the important difference between those that produced the cold and those that did not is that one group was susceptible to it whilst the other one was not. Plainly the dose of bugs is a factor too. Nevertheless, some of those who were very close to the man would not get ill despite receiving a very large dose of bugs and some, who were in the most distant part of the bus, would catch it despite receiving a small dose.

What is susceptibility?

In order to become ill one has to be susceptible to that illness. If a person is not susceptible to an illness then he (or she) simply will not develop it. So when did all those people on the bus who went down with a cold become ill? When did the illness actually begin? We commonly think of the illness as the symptoms but I would ask you to expand your view of disease to take into consideration the individual's susceptibility because, as we have just seen, it is essential to the process of producing an illness that he be susceptible to it. With that in mind, how can we reasonably leave it out of our picture of disease?

When we consider the essential role of susceptibility it becomes plain that the people who caught a cold in the bus were 'ill' before they ever stepped onto it, for if they had been healthy they would never have picked up the bugs in the first place. How long they had been 'carrying' their susceptibility to that cold around with them just waiting to meet up with the right bugs will depend upon the individual circumstances of each of them.

At this point there is a need to distinguish between two uses of the word disease (or illness). Commonly we consider a disease to be the symptoms that we experience when ill but if we are to take the susceptibility into account then we need a word to include it in this larger view of disease. Unfortunately, we have no such word in the English language. When the word disease is used in the field of Homoeopathy it often should be understood to include the susceptibility and it should be apparent from the context when this is so.

You may consider the susceptibility as the soil in which the seeds of disease are sown. If the soil is not right then the seeds will not grow. The seeds are all the external influences that tend to throw us out of balance and they may affect us on any level of our being; on the physical level it may be something simple like being exposed to a cold wind, getting soaked in the rain or even some form of trauma. They will all tend to put a stress on the system and depending on our health or susceptibility we will be affected to a greater or a lesser degree. On the emotional level, stresses come in many different forms; such as problems in relationships, with family or the grief from the death of a loved one. On the mental level we may experience stresses from business problems and financial worries, the pressure of examinations and so on. Frequently the stresses involve a combination of these different levels.

Natural healing powers

Our natural healing or life powers will cope with many of these stresses without ever producing any symptoms. It is as if our vitality is sufficient to stop those apparently unhelpful influences from having any effect. A point may be reached when the external stresses on any level become so great that in order to defend, repair and maintain order in the system the healing powers produce symptoms and signs of what we call an illness or disease. If our vitality is low then our susceptibility is high.

The body has an organising intelligence that orders it and runs all the processes and functions of the parts and integrates them into the whole. It operates through the agencies of the different control systems such as the autonomic nervous system, hormonal system, immune system etc. Without this intelligence the body would rapidly cease to exist. This same intelligence is concerned with the natural healing power of the body. Is it sensible to consider that this natural intelligence or healing power would produce a situation that was without a purpose, for which no reason existed and which was harmful to the person **when considered as a whole?** It may cause damage to a part of the person but we should not lose sight of the whole person if we wish to understand what is going on.

What is the purpose of symptoms?

What, then, is the purpose of disease symptoms? Is it not likely that the healing powers are continually trying to maintain order in the system but once the external stresses reach a certain level this can no longer be done 'passively' but the very attempt to keep a balance produces outward signs which we generally find uncomfortable and so call disease; which is literally a lack of ease or disease. Viewed in this way the symptoms and signs of disease appear entirely different. They are no longer the inconvenient, unwanted, useless and 'why did I have to get it now' things that they are commonly thought to be but they are actually the manifestation of each person's attempt to get well, to maintain order and balance in the system. They are the external effect of the internal fight to get well, recover and heal. They are not a part of becoming ill, which went on, generally unnoticed, beforehand, but are a part of the healing process.

Now it becomes a little clearer why, in a young healthy child where 'disease' serves its function in its most simple and natural form, it has been observed that the child is more well after an acute ailment has resolved than he was before it started. It also becomes quite understandable why people tend to become 'ill' when there are a lot of stresses going on in their lives and especially at times of life crises such as griefs, changes in work and divorce. Quite simply, these are times when there is more healing to be done, more effort is required by the natural healing powers to maintain order or to put it slightly differently, it is no longer possible for a balance and harmony to be sustained without the production of symptoms of disease.

A further question may have arisen; why is the fertile soil or the susceptibility present in the first place? What gave rise to it? This is connected to questions about why some people are born with poor health and touches on some very deep aspects of philosophy which I will not attempt to discuss in this book. Suffice it to say that some people are better built at the beginning. They are constructed with few weaknesses and have a sound, strong constitution. These are the people who are often quoted as enjoying good health to a ripe old age despite smoking, drinking and never taking any exercise. These days there are not many of them around.

The key to understanding Homoeopathy

How does Homoeopathy fit into this picture of disease? Once it is understood that the symptoms of disease are actually a good thing in that they are the highly characteristic outward indication of the healing and balancing process that is going on inside each individual person, then to give a medicine that is capable of mimicking and bringing about that same process suddenly seems to be a good idea; both totally reasonable and logical.

The key to Homoeopathy is that no two people suffer from the same disease. We each have our own highly individual ways of reacting to the stresses of life and of maintaining our inner harmony. Certainly there are broad similarities and a degree of categorisation is possible but with detailed analysis there are always differences. After all, no two people are exactly the same, at least none that I have heard of or met!

Take as an example a simple sore throat. Let us assume that we have selected twenty cases who all have the same bugs growing in their throats. The usual view is that they are all suffering from the same disease and yet it is plain that there are marked differences between the reaction of one patient to that of another. For instance one may find marked relief from taking warm drinks which would make another feel much worse; one may have a high fever and sweats whilst another has no fever at all; one may be hot and want to be uncovered and in the fresh air whilst another is hot yet wants to be covered up to his chin; one may wish to continue his work whilst another might only wish to lie down and die and so on.

These differences are an indication of the unique way in which each individual is responding to the circumstances in which he finds himself and of the state of that person as a whole, that is they show how his healing powers are operating at that time.

Now, if a medicine is given to a healthy person and it causes them to produce a particular reaction, a set of symptoms, then these symptoms are the healing response that this particular medicine is capable of bringing about. To put it another way, bearing in mind that symptoms are part of the healing process and not the disease process, then particular medicines will bring about particular healing responses, that is symptoms.

Like cures like

It now makes perfect sense to give a remedy that is capable of bringing about the same or very similar healing responses, that is symptoms, to the healing response which is occurring in the patient as shown by his individual symptoms. Hence we have the Law of Similars which is very ancient and predates the formulation of Homoeopathy in the eighteenth century. It was known to Paracelsus in the fifteenth century, it can be found in the fourth century BC in Hippocratic writings and is one of the principles of treatment in Ayurvedic Medicine which was written down over 5000 years ago. It states – 'that which can cause a disease can also cure it' or 'like cures like'. It is interesting that examples of this law in operation are found in many different areas. In the field of cancer therapy it is well known that irradiation can cause tumours and yet they can also be treated by radiation and many of the drugs used in chemotherapy for tumours can also cause tumours. Digitoxin can cause heart irregularities, or arrhythmias, but it is also very useful in the treatment of certain arrhythmias. There are many others.

Many of these seemingly contradictory properties of the agents are related to dose. The healthier a person is, the higher the dose necessary to throw that person out of balance, as shown by the appearance of symptoms and signs. In disease, even a small stimulus, if it is aligned with the healing process of the individual, will have an effect. Nevertheless, a higher dose or one not sufficiently matched to the individual will still tend to overstimulate and may then cause what are usually called side-effects. The closer the stimulus or medicine is aligned to the healing in the patient the lower the dose of drug needed; they are more susceptible to it. The unwanted effects, which are an indication of the mis-match between the powers of the drug and those of the patient either in quality (the type of medicine used) or in quantity (the dose administered), are fewer.

This explains a phenomenon frequently observed in Homoeopathy; often after the administration of the indicated remedy there is a brief and mild worsening of the symptoms followed by their gradual resolution. This is due to the stimulus of the remedy causing the healing powers to respond. In principle if the dose were to exactly meet the requirements of the patient there would be no observable reaction before the resolution took place. In practice this rarely happens and a mild reaction is commonly produced.

It can be seen that the correct dose of the correct medicine will aid a person's healing. Give too much and it may bring about the very conditions it is capable of curing; 'Through the like, disease is produced and through the application of the like it is cured', said Hippocrates over 2000 years ago.

Homoeopathy is why a remedy is given, not what is given

It is well known that Homoeopathic remedies are very dilute in their preparation though their effects cannot be explained so simply. For those that understand such terminology it might be said that the remedies work at the level of energy and not of matter. Here we again begin to approach the deeper aspects of philosophy and I do not intend to say any more about it here. The method of preparation of the remedies and how they act is not essential to an understanding of Homoeopathy. Homoeopathy is about why a remedy is given, not what is given.

There is a great deal of nonsense spoken about Homoeopathy that stems from this basic misconception. So often we hear about a Homoeopathic remedy for colds or flu or arthritis etc. Only a little thought will show what a nonsense this is, for, as we have just seen, no two individuals manifest their illnesses in exactly the same way even if they are given the same disease label. So how can there be one 'Homoeopathic' remedy to suit everyone with that 'disease'? Plainly it has nothing to do with Homoeopathy which is concerned with individualisation. It is only when a substance is matched with a patient according to the Law of Similars that it becomes Homoeopathic. When it is sitting in the medicine chest or pharmacy it is not Homoeopathic at all; it is just a potentised remedy (potentisation is the name given to the process of preparation of the remedies used). Potentised remedies are used in many different forms of therapy, not just Homoeopathy. They can even be used allopathically (as in orthodox medicine) and this is just what is happening in the situation above when one or two remedies are advocated for the treatment of everyone with one disease label.

It is worthy of note at this point that the decision as to what is the correct or most similar remedy for a patient is not necessarily simple or straightforward. In acute diseases it is generally adequate to look only at the symptoms of the acute disease itself. How the person is being affected as a whole is usually quite clear and obvious. In constitutional treatment, a much greater insight into what is happening and the significance of the symptoms is required, that is as to what constitutes the totality of the disease for which a most similar remedy is required. This is why, as has been said earlier, conditions which more closely reflect the constitutional state of the person should only be treated by experienced therapists and not the well intentioned novice.

The remedy pictures

How is the capability of each remedy known? How is the picture which determines its use ascertained? Very simply by giving the remedy to a group of healthy people in a carefully controlled and closely monitored fashion. All the changes and symptoms that arise are noted and studied to detect patterns and trends that are characteristic and commonly occur. These are likely to be of great importance when prescribing the remedy for a patient. This process is called a Proving of the remedy and strict criteria are laid down in order to ensure that the true action of the remedy is brought out and not any interferences from other sources. A properly conducted Proving may last for many months.

Once the Proving picture is obtained then enough is known about the remedy to start using it in practice. Subsequently, when the remedy is given to treat sick people, other symptoms that had not been brought out in the Proving are noted to be cured by the remedy and if this happens repeatedly then those symptoms are added to the picture of that remedy. So gradually a fuller understanding of the actions of the remedies is obtained enabling them to be used with greater accuracy. This process has continued from one generation of Homoeopaths to the next so that instead of the new discoveries sweeping away all the previous ideas, as commonly occurs in many 'scientific' studies, the knowledge of remedies, known as Materia Medica, is continually being added to, developed and refined.

The holistic approach

How is the progress of a patient assessed? In Homoeopathy and many other types of alternative medicine the patient's illness is placed in a much larger context. The susceptibility has already been spoken of but the assessment of a patient involves looking at their health on all levels, including physical, mental and emotional. Since there is an intelligent system at work in each person it follows that if discomfort or dysfunction is necessary in order to maintain harmony within the system as a whole then the disease will manifest in the least important parts possible thus preserving the higher functions of the person for as long as possible. Therefore, it becomes apparent that there is a hierarchy of symptoms and disease.

Among the most important functions are the mental faculties without which a person could no longer lead a useful life. It takes little thought to see that someone who is physically crippled and confined to a wheelchair may still lead a very full life if his mental and higher faculties are in good order whereas a physically fit but totally demented person has little left to give and little capacity to receive except for physical care and a little love. Their life could certainly not be described as full.

Within each realm there is a hierarchy, so in very general terms in the physical sphere a skin rash or a cold is of minor significance whereas a heart, lung or brain disease is much more serious. Diseases of joints, muscles and gut lie somewhere in the middle. In the emotional field, minor anger and irritability are less deep than fears and phobias and mentally, a little forgetfulness is less significant than delusions or confusional states.

This is a very brief view of the type of assessment that is made during constitutional treatment. The focus of a patient's illness, in relation to the hierarchy, is assessed and monitored. To be sure that a patient is truly regaining their health, it is of no value just to know that the symptoms of his complaint have been relieved, rather the focus of his disease has to be seen to be shifting into less important areas, that is, moving down the hierarchy. If someone 'recovers' from their arthritic condition but later develops a heart condition then, in reality, they never recovered at all but the focus of their disease shifted from a more superficial to a deeper level. Such connections are occasionally recognised in orthodox medicine where there is not a long time delay between one complaint developing and the next, though the significance of the link between diseases is frequently missed.

For example it is well known that asthma and eczema are linked but what is frequently overlooked is the way that a person's asthma can be bad at a time when their eczema is quiet and their eczema can be its worst when the asthma is quiet. This natural sequence of events is frequently obscured when the condition is treated without taking the constitution into account.

The Law of Cure

With a view to aiding the assessment of a patient's progress there are a few simple guidelines that can be followed; for cure to be taking place the disease should go from within to without, from organs of greater importance to lesser importance, from above to below and to disappear in the reverse order to their original appearance. The last is probably the most important since it has been observed time and again that, during constitutional treatment, old symptoms reminiscent of previous states of health tend to recur, until a state of health can sometimes eventually be achieved where the only illnesses experienced are those common to childhood, such as coughs, colds, sore throats and skin rashes. For many reasons this cannot be attained by all patients though most can be helped some of the way back, to former states of better health.

Finally

This is a very brief overview of some of the aspects of Homoeopathy and a view of the world which may help to shed a little light on what is happening with a person's health. This book does not aim to be a comprehensive text covering the philosophy and principles of Homoeopathy; it is a practical book designed to be used by anyone wishing to treat the common acute illnesses, particularly those occurring during childhood. A complete understanding of the theory and philosophy is not necessary in order to use Homoeopathy effectively and safely in these types of condition. However a little knowledge of the philosophy is useful and may stimulate an interest. Whether or not what has been suggested here reflects your view of the world is immaterial. If this book helps in the selection of remedies to assist the natural healing process then it will have achieved its purpose. This selection is not difficult and requires no academic training. The ability to observe is of far greater importance and is readily enhanced by practice.

When it comes to the treatment of chronic and recurrent illnesses such as those listed in the section *Conditions Requiring Constitutional Therapy* on page 137, the situation is quite different. If the condition is a recurrent one such as migraine or period pains, it is perfectly possible to use a book like this to find remedies that will give relief each time the pain occurs but it will not prevent the pain recurring next time. Curative treatment for such conditions is quite beyond the scope of this book. They reflect processes taking place much more deeply within the individual and are dependent upon many factors such as constitutional make-up, heredity, diet, life events, lifestyle, environment and so on. Anyone requiring therapy for such conditions would be well advised to seek out an experienced practitioner in whichever constitutional therapy best suits their individual needs. Individualisation is common to all the reputable therapies of which I am aware and that includes the choice of therapy itself.

There is much more to discover and there are many methods of discovery. Homoeopathy is not the only practice that uses the concepts presented here and no one of repute, of whom I am aware, would claim that Homoeopathy has all the answers or that it will suit everyone. It certainly has something of value to offer and there is only one way to find out whom it will suit; try it!

§2 How to use Homoeopathy in practice

The aim

The essence of Homoeopathy is to match a remedy picture to the disease picture in an individual. A picture in this sense consists of the collection of symptoms which characterise the remedy or the patient with his illness. Symptoms are changes from the normal state of a person occurring at any level of his being and would range from changes of mood or behaviour to physical things like pains, temperature reactions, colour changes, sweats etc.

That which a remedy is capable of causing (that is, the picture of the remedy) is also able to be cured by that remedy. This is the Law of Similars – 'like cures like'. An explanation of why this should be is given in Chapter 1. However, Homoeopathy can be used for simple acute illnesses such as those described in this book, without a full understanding of its philosophy and theory. Remember the aim – to find the remedy with the most similar picture to the picture of disease in the patient.

Here arises the first problem: how completely must the picture of the disease and the remedy match in order to be assured of a beneficial result?

Clearly, the more complete the fit between the remedy and the illness the more certain and the greater will be the success of the prescription. Only an expert after much study and practical experience will achieve consistently good responses. So how can the beginner maximise the chance of success? It was with this in mind that the book was written. Some of the most important features of the remedies are highlighted and the information is presented in an easy-to-use tabular form. It gives additional information which can be used as experience grows and by those who already possess some knowledge of Homoeopathy. It is designed to enable anyone to make a start in finding, with a reasonable degree of accuracy, remedies to treat common illnesses and, as time goes on, to develop a knowledge and understanding of the remedies and their uses.

The book is designed to bridge the gap between the very simple and inadequate descriptions of use given with many Homoeopathic remedies and the much larger texts, the depth and complexity of which would put Homoeopathy quite beyond all but the most dedicated of beginners.

The method

Firstly, the picture of the disease in the patient is needed. The process of obtaining this information is called 'taking the case'.

Taking the case

There are only two requirements when taking a case and they are interdependent: **Observation** with all the senses and **objectivity** or freedom from interpretation of what is observed.

Observation

Observation involves seeing, hearing, smelling, touching and, rarely, tasting! The vital clue to an individual's sickness may come through any of the senses, so use them all. Having observed something, just record it and do not reason it out as to why it is so. Best of all, record the patient's own words, especially for the important symptoms. The less thinking and interpreting that goes on the better. By all means make enquiries in order to aid observation. Indeed, the largest part of the case will be heard as the patient tells of his symptoms except, of course, in the case of an infant.

Keep a record

You may like to keep a family or personal health record to note all relevant health matters – patterns of health, details of specific illnesses, their treatment and outcome, accidents, vaccinations and their effect etc. It would be interesting to note also the stresses that occur from time to time, be they physical, mental or emotional and to observe their effect on health. This can sometimes be quite enlightening! One of the secrets of staying healthy is to discover what it is that tends to throw you out of balance and causes illnesses to appear. This will be very individual and may be important for your long term health. It is good to regain a healthy state. It is far better to never get unhealthy in the first place!

When taking a case, even your own, write it down in whatever layout and form you find suits you. You may divide it into sections, such as in the tables, record it just as it is spoken, or however else you wish, but do record it for later reference and to help you learn.

What to observe

Allow the patient to speak of what they notice to be wrong with themselves and try not to put words into the patient's mouth. Use questions such as 'what else?, what more?, can you tell me more about that?' in order to extract more information.

What the patient tells you without prompting will usually be of greater importance. Of course you have to take into account the basic personality of the patient; some will tell all without needing to be questioned, others need tact, diplomacy and perseverance to get any symptoms from them. Sometimes it can be as hard a task as pulling teeth from a hungry crocodile but do not despair! This fact in itself may be a symptom of the illness, particularly if it is not usual for them to behave in that way. This would be an example of a mental symptom. The more marked the change in behaviour or mental state, the more important it will be to find a remedy with that same mental picture.

Underline anything that is very prominent and strong. You may wish to underline some things two or three times. Make a special note of anything that is unexpected such as a sore throat that is better for swallowing solid food – normally one would expect this to make it worse. Another example would be a fever with a dry mouth but no thirst. Symptoms like this are called strange, rare and *peculiar*, and are often of prime importance in finding the remedy or group of remedies from which to make one's selection.

Other things to be observed would be the patient's appearance, presence or absence of heat and sweat in different areas of the body, his behaviour and mood, what he wants in his surroundings and environment, does he want to be still or moving, if he moves why does he move, does he want fresh air or to be covered, or both, or neither, and so on!

Refer to the tables for ideas

A brief look at the tables will give you an idea of the type of symptoms and detail that is required. After the patient has run out of things to tell you on his own initiative make enquiries into each of the sections covering the particular complaint of the patient. Ask for details of sensations, where they are situated, where they move to, how they start and change, find out what the pattern is but take care to use open ended questions whenever possible; questions that cannot be answered by a simple 'yes' or 'no', such as 'How does your head feel?' instead of 'Do you have a headache?'

Be sure to ask about the *modalities* of the symptoms – these are the factors which make it better (>) or worse (<). For brevity it is worth using these little symbols which are easy to learn. As can be seen from the tables, just about anything may affect a symptom. The stronger, more definite and consistent it is, the more important it will be as a symptom of the case.

Under *Cause and Onset* look at what has been happening in the preceding hours or days to the onset of the illness and consider the speed with which the illness came on and the order of events. Causes might range from becoming wet or chilled, a change in the weather, overexertion, dietary indiscretions etc. to emotional factors such as grief or anger.

Do not ignore these emotional factors as triggers of illness. That headaches can follow arguments and diarrhoea may appear in anticipation of some unusual event is well known but the role that the emotions play in many if not most illnesses is rarely appreciated.

In general if an illness has appeared rapidly and vigorously over a matter of hours then one should look for a cause in the preceding few hours or day at the most. If it appears slowly with a few days warning of something being not quite right and the patient gradually sinks into the illness, then the cause is likely to lie several days or even a week earlier. It may reflect some prolonged period of stress at any level of being; physical, mental or emotional. Whilst first aid remedies may be of use for each episode of acute illness, proper constitutional treatment and advice is likely to be more appropriate to help with the long term tendency to become unwell repeatedly.

Under the section of *Abdominal Conditions* it will be noticed that there are three lots of modalities. These relate to each of the preceding sections, that is the modalities of the sensation, the modalities of the diarrhoea, and the modalities of the nausea and vomiting.

Concomitant symptoms are symptoms not directly related to but arising at the same time as, the main complaint such as a headache with diarrhoea or cold sores with a fever – things which are repeatedly associated, so that the patient might say 'Whenever I get this problem I always get a stomach upset' or whatever it may be.

The final section of the tables is headed *Mentals and Generals*. Mental symptoms relate to the mood, behaviour, speech pattern etc. of the patient. Characteristics of the patient when well that are still present when ill are not actually a part of the picture of the acute illness and are therefore **not** important when selecting a remedy for the acute disease. This actually applies to any symptom, not just to mental conditions. Whereas if someone who is normally very placid and kind became ill, say with an earache and at the same time became irritable and bad tempered, then this would be a highly significant symptom. That patient would need a remedy capable of causing just such an irritability. Mental symptoms arising in this way are generally of the greatest importance when selecting the most similar remedy.

General symptoms are symptoms that relate to the whole person in general and not just to the particular site of the problem. So if a person had a sore throat and it burned, this burning would be a particular symptom because it was limited to a single focus of his illness. If on the other hand he also had some burning when he passed a motion, his feet burned at night and his eyes were dry and burning, then it is clear that the sensation of 'burning' runs throughout many areas of the person's body and so becomes characteristic of him as a whole, that is, it becomes General.

General symptoms can be preceded by the words 'I am', as in 'I am thirsty, hot, tired, lacking energy or burning all over'. The opposite of a general symptom is a particular symptom. This relates only to an isolated part of the person and is usually preceded by the word 'my', such as 'my head hurts, my throat is dry', etc. Things which affect the person as a whole are of much greater importance than those affecting only a part. So mental and general symptoms carry greater weight when evaluating a case.

More information on Mentals and Generals is given in the Materia Medica section towards the end of the book, which covers the most commonly required remedies.

This guide will help you to take the case. Bear in mind that in order to find the most similar remedy we need to have symptoms that mark out how one individual's illness differs from another's. We need the symptoms that characterise the individuality of the disease process in each case. So symptoms that are common and occur in most or all cases of that type of complaint are useless when selecting a remedy, for example, nausea worse for eating, pains worse for touching the sore part, dry mouth with thirst.

Likewise symptoms that are indefinite, mild and nebulous. Unless, of course, all the symptoms are like that in which case it becomes a general symptom and might point towards a remedy like *Ferrum phos.* or maybe *Pulsatilla*.

So look out for the strong, the peculiar, the characteristic symptoms, any general symptoms that run through the case in different areas of the body and any changes in the mental state of the patient. Make sure that you have all the details of each symptom: any cause, the speed of onset, the site, the sensations, the modalities etc. Have you ascertained the strength and consistency of each symptom? This will help you to appreciate the unique state of the patient and just how the illness is affecting him.

There is no one way to take a case. It is a creative and individual process reflecting the relationship between yourself and the patient. This is why you should be as free from emotional upset and involvement as possible when taking it.

There is only one way to become proficient at anything – practice! In that practice you will discover different ways of obtaining the information to suit the different types of cases. They will, of course, also suit your own character and style of doing things.

Case analysis and use of the tables

Now that you have 'taken the case' it needs to be analysed. When selecting the most important features of the case they should be clear, strong and characteristic of the patient's illness right now. Be quite sure the symptoms are new changes and do not relate to the patient's normal state of health. Changes of intensity may be included though proportionally less significance can be given to them.

Much has already been said to help you evaluate the importance of each symptom. The evaluation mainly arises from a combination of three factors. Firstly the depth of the symptom – that is at what level of the person's being it is taking place, secondly the strength of the symptom and thirdly how uniquely characteristic is the symptom of the patient's state.

A useful guide to the first two is to see what effect a symptom has on the patient's ability to function as a whole, creative, happy, loving human being, taking into account their normal state of course! It is clear that anything which affects the mind will be of prime importance in this (see Chapter 1) as also will be anything that affects the person as a whole. Mental and General symptoms are therefore ranked high.

Particular symptoms which relate to the separate parts are usually of less significance. Nevertheless if the patient is mentally and emotionally unaffected but has, for example, a pain somewhere, then the details of the pain will make up the whole case, or 'totality' as it is called, for which a similar remedy must be found. This can also happen if a pain is very severe and strong such that it makes all the other symptoms pale into insignificance.

Peculiar symptoms, also called 'Strange, Rare and *Peculiar* symptoms', fall outside this method of evaluation because they may be very debilitating or make little difference to the patient's ability to function. Their high ranking stems from the individuality of the symptom to that patient. If the Peculiar is also strong and consistent then this will increase its importance even occasionally to the point where it will override Mental and General symptoms when evaluating the case. Peculiars are by definition uncommon but they are worth searching for and if present in a case would strongly favour any remedies showing that same symptom. Examples of Peculiar symptoms would be 'dry mouth without thirst', 'burning pain better for (>) heat', 'symptoms affecting one half of the body only'.

Clearly the strength of each symptom needs to be taken into account. The way in which the patient speaks of his symptoms, his tone of voice, choice of language, gestures and expressions will all tell of the intensity.

At first you may like to employ a points system to help in your evaluation of symptoms, though with practice and familiarity this will not be necessary:

Mentals are worth 3 points.

Physical symptoms that are Generals (symptoms that can be expressed 'I am . . .') are worth 2 points.

Particular symptoms that relate to the separate parts of the body are worth 1 point.

Peculiars might come anywhere depending on their degree of peculiarity. The more that you know about what is normal and expected in diseases the easier it will be to evaluate the Peculiars. Most of it is just common sense.

The ranking of the modalities and concomitants relates to the individual symptoms concerned and should fall into one of the above categories.

Finally, having ranked the symptoms as above, additional points need to be allocated according to the strength of each symptom on a scale of 1 to 3. Take into account the intensity and consistency in deciding how many points to give for this.

The sum of these two numbers together will allow you to choose the most important and characteristic symptoms of the case which should be used for the next step.

Selecting the remedy

The main area or areas of complaint will indicate the first tables to consider. Note the selection headings for these areas and write down the most important features of the case that occur in each of these sections in a layout that will make the next step easy for you.

Look along the sections of the tables and match the main features of the case with the features of the remedies. The remedy picture may include a lot of other symptoms that are not in the case itself. Do not worry about this so long as all or most of the important symptoms of the case are in the remedy. Construct a list of matching remedies.

The first two pages for each set of tables contains the remedies most frequently indicated. The remedies have been grouped for easier comparison and so do not appear alphabetically.

If you find that none are a good match then you are probably including too much detail and are not just selecting the most important features. Go back to the case and review critically the main characteristic symptoms eliminating those that are not strong, are vague, have perhaps only occurred once or twice and are not really important features of the illness. Consider using the points system to help you.

If you find six or more remedies are matching then you have probably included too many common symptoms. These you will recall are the ones that are characteristic of the disease in general in everyone and not the disease in the individual. You should also review the case looking for the more individual features in it. It may be necessary to return to the patient and ask for more details of symptoms and search for any important features that have been overlooked.

Ideally you should end up with less than six and probably more than one or two remedies to consider in greater detail in the tables.

The second stage in the selection process is to refine the match. Is there a remedy picture which most closely resembles the important features of the case? Do many or most of the important symptoms of the remedy which appear in bold type match the strongest symptoms of the case? Are the more minor symptoms of the case to be found in the remedy? This is of less importance but may confirm what was already clear or it may help to differentiate between two or more remedies which are equally close.

Read the whole case again, read all the symptoms of the remedy and refer to the Materia Medica of the most common remedies at the back of the book for the final comparison which does not rely on the numerical evaluation.

You may find that reference to more than one set of tables will help you. For instance someone with a sore throat may well also have a fever and you will get a fuller picture by looking at the remedies in both sections.

When comparing the symptoms of the case and the remedy you should also note that the most important symptoms do not clash or contradict. For example *Belladonna* has a rapid, vigorous and violent fever coming on quickly. If the patient's fever took several days to appear then it is much less likely to be *Belladonna* no matter how much the rest of the picture looks like it. You will also find that some remedies have opposite symptoms, for example *Belladonna* may be thirstless or thirsty in its fever. Both pictures may occur. If one is very much more common and prominent than the other then it will be written in bold type and the other in ordinary type.

A warning should be issued here. You almost never find all the symptoms of the case in a remedy picture and you will never find all the symptoms of a remedy in the disease picture of the case, so do not look for it or try to fit it all in. It will only exasperate you! It is much more important to look out for those strong, peculiar, characteristic symptoms and any mental or general symptoms. Let those be your guide when selecting the remedy.

For the absolute beginner and those who lack the time or enthusiasm, the selection of a remedy can take place by considering primarily the very important symptoms of the remedies which have been printed in bold type, ignoring all the information in ordinary type.

Different ways of selecting the remedy

Selecting a remedy is part science, part art. Commonly it starts off being a scientific process, evaluating and carefully comparing all the different features of the case with the most likely remedies. This tends to be the way that the gentlemen work it out. They are generally more logical, step by step, and scientific in their approach to a problem.

The artistic approach involves a more intuitive, creative way of thinking that is not always entirely logical, is found more often in the ladies' approach and comes with experience. This is also a valid way and can produce better results than the scientific way of working. It does require a certain knowledge of the remedies, though. Commonly the prescriber will be fairly familiar with the remedies and will 'just know' the remedy as the case is taken or may only need to look up one or two symptoms to confirm the remedy.

The process of evaluating and matching symptom pictures as a whole, which takes place in this more intuitive process, might be compared to the difference between a mathematician and a child when presented with a simple sum such as 4 + 3. The child will work it out on his fingers and get the right answer. The mathematician will look at it and simply know the answer. Both are right but one is quicker. However, once upon a time the mathematician was a child too.

This process must not be confused with guessing or wishful thinking. It is very different, and as you can see has to be based on some knowledge or understanding. As this knowledge of the remedies grows in you, do not be surprised if you sometimes 'just know' which is the right remedy and know it without any doubts. Sometimes there is something about the 'image' of a remedy which just seems to fit the patient. Have a good look at that remedy and see if your intuitive feelings can be justified.

However you work in selecting a remedy find the way that suits you and gives you results as shown by a good response to its administration. The accuracy of your selection can only be proved by giving the remedy and the patient getting better. In this sense every Homoeopathic prescription is an experiment, even those of the most experienced professional!

Plenty of spaces have been left throughout the book on which you can add your own notes about the remedies. Only add those things of which you are quite sure. If there is a doubt put it in pencil and wait for confirmation from your own experience or from the reports of others.

Which potency?

The more a remedy is potentised, the quicker and deeper its action. It also becomes more specific and for the higher potencies the remedy selection has to be more accurate for the remedy to work.

Low potencies are usually regarded as being those up to and including the 30c or 30x. The letters 'c' and 'x' refer to the dilution factor used in the preparation of the remedy and it need not concern us here, as to all practical intents and purposes for home prescribing the difference is negligible. Commonly one can readily obtain the following potencies; 6x, 6c, 12x, 12c, 30x and 30c. The higher the number the greater the potency of the remedy.

For the conditions described in this book it is the selection of the remedy that is of far greater importance than the specific potency used. As a general rule if the sick person requires a remedy and you only have it available in one potency then that is the correct potency no matter what it is!

If you are going to stock your medicine cupboard with only one potency of each remedy, my personal choice would be 12x or 12c. This will go a little further than a 6 but is not quite so specific as a 30. If you have built up some experience using the remedies then you will find the 30 an excellent potency for acute illness. If you are new to Homoeopathy and do not intend to follow case taking and evaluation guidelines, such as have been given in this chapter, then a set of 6x remedies will serve you best.

In the vast majority of cases the 6th potency will work just as well as the 30th and does not require such accuracy. One point that may help you is that the lower the potency the more frequently it is likely to need repeating.

Safety and Storage

Having selected a remedy it must now be given, but first I would like to put in a little reassurance.

What if it is the wrong one? In treating acute illnesses there are only two outcomes to giving the wrong low potency remedy. Firstly, there may be a partial response which does not last long, and secondly, there may be no response at all. In order to bring about a deterioration in the patient's condition with low potency remedies one would have to keep on repeating the wrong remedy many times and even then it is unlikely that much would happen unless the patient were particularly frail and weak, in which case they should be having constitutional treatment to boost their overall state and not 'first aid' treatment for the little bits that go wrong. Someone who has much chronic ill health should not be treated except by an experienced practitioner. Nevertheless it is very difficult to do any harm with 'first aid' Homoeopathy using low potency remedies. They are very safe.

Even if a child took a whole bottle full of remedies it would not be harmed! This is because the important factor is the frequency of repetition of the remedy and not the quantity given. No more than one pill at a time is needed and the effect is not stronger by giving a full bottle. It is rather like having a door handle to be opened. In the opening of a door it matters not if the strong hand of a weight lifter turns the knob or the delicate hand of a lady, the effect is the same. The door is opened. So it is with Homoeopathy, the quantity does not matter, it is the quality that is important.

During pregnancy low potency remedies can be taken for acute illnesses without risk to mother or child.

The pills themselves, if stored tightly capped, out of the sun and away from strong smells, can be kept for years without loss of potency. Keep them in their original containers and if you need to transfer them make sure they go into a new, labelled bottle or clean paper envelope. **Never** reuse old remedy bottles or envelopes for a different remedy or potency.

Only open one remedy bottle at a time.

Although they are much safer than allopathic or conventional drugs it is obviously advisable to store them in a safe place, out of reach of little fingers.

How do you give the remedy?

The remedy may come as a liquid potency when the dose is one drop, as granules when the dose is 10 or 20 grains (like sugar grains or the 'hundreds and thousands' used to decorate cakes) or, most commonly as tablets when the dose is one tablet.

Rules

1. Do not touch the pills. The patient himself may pick one up with clean hands, but no one else. You may also use a clean spoon or piece of paper.

2. Do not return pills to the stock bottle if accidentally tipped out. Discard them.

3. Suck the pill under the tongue. They are made from sugar and should easily dissolve. If it is slow, crush it with the teeth and then suck the pieces under the tongue.

4. Ideally the mouth should be clean with no flavours, food or drink for 10 or 15 minutes before or after taking the pill.

5. Whilst treating anyone with remedies they should avoid anything with a strong smell, scent, aroma or perfume. No aromatic oils, vapour rubs, smelly nasal decongestants like menthol or eucalyptus etc. Some Homoeopaths will also advise avoiding coffee and toothpaste; others will not. You may suit yourself on that one! What I do is to stop these last two if apparently indicated remedies are not working as well as I would have expected. It is a good thing to stop coffee anyway from a general health point of view but the benefits of this would only be apparent from a long term change, not just for a few days.

Children can either take remedies as a powder by crushing the pill between two clean teaspoons, or dissolved in a little clean, fresh water in a glass.

Plussing

In a very acute illness the remedy may need to be repeated every hour or two at first until sustained improvement sets in. In this situation it is often worth dissolving two or three tablets, or their equivalent, in a clean glass of fresh water and taking a teaspoonful when needed. Between doses the water is best agitated by lifting a spoonful up in the air and allowing it to splash back in the glass ten or twenty times. This is called plussing and it slightly alters the potency of the remedy in the glass which helps to maintain its effectiveness.

After the first prescription

The rule here is not to repeat or change the remedy until the action of the previous dose has ceased. This may mean a lot of waiting!

One of four things commonly happens:

1. The patient gets better. Do not repeat the remedy whilst improvement is still occurring. Nothing more to be done!

2. The symptoms get slightly worse straight after the remedy is given. This is a common reaction to the effect of the remedy and you should wait and

expect to see an improvement over the next few minutes or an hour or so depending on how severe the illness is. The more vigorous and acute the illness is the quicker things change. So in a lingering slow fever you might wait several hours for a response to a remedy, whereas in a delirious, high, raging fever one would expect to see changes within ten or fifteen minutes.

3. The patient improves for a time, say an hour or more, then either stops getting better and the picture becomes more or less static, or begins to slip back again with the same symptoms. Your prescription has worked and now is the time to repeat the same remedy.

4. No effect. Often the first change is that the patient begins to feel better in himself but still has all the symptoms. This is a very important sign of a good response and must not be overlooked. You should wait and look for other improvements to follow.

If there has really been no response, wait for a time depending on the vigour and severity of the illness (see para. 2). If no changes occur then repeat the same remedy and wait again. Do this once or twice more before giving up on that remedy. If there is no response after three or four pills then either the prescription is wrong or the remedy is no good and has lost its potency for some reason. If you are a beginner it is a fair bet that the prescription is not right and you should review the case and select another remedy.

If you have some experience and would have expected the remedy to work then put a pencil dot or mark on the bottle. If you find next time you need that remedy that it again does not work, put another mark on the bottle and give it one more chance before discarding the whole bottle. Very occasionally a bottle will become contaminated and lose its potency. Do remember to rub out your dots if a remedy works at a later date and only mark your bottle when the remedy has no effect if you are very certain that it should have worked.

Often changes are marked and obvious, there being no doubt as what to do. Sometimes when the changes are slower it can be more difficult because allowance has to be made for the natural variations that occur hour by hour in an illness even without any treatment. Here it is important to remember the point made in paragraph 2 above; vigorous, severe illnesses respond to remedies in a vigorous way. They also tend to 'use up' remedies quickly which may need repeating several times an hour at first but always according to the changes in the symptom picture. Cases of this severity are likely to be the ones which would lead you to seek expert medical advice from your local health care practitioner. Whilst you are waiting for the expert help to arrive, there is no reason why you should not take the person's case and find a remedy for him. Even whilst a person is waiting to go to hospital there may be something you can do to help.

Very often the more severe and acute the illness, the clearer the disease picture so that the similar remedy may actually be easier to select. If the picture is clear, give the remedy. If you follow the guidelines given in this book it can only help and certainly will not harm.

Slow lingering illnesses may require only one remedy a day or less. The patient will tell you by his symptoms what needs to be done, when to wait and when to treat.

As a rough guide the 'average' illness that will put a person in bed is likely to need a remedy between 3 and 8 times a day, needing more at the beginning of the illness than later on. A less severe cough, cold, throat or stomach upset etc. may need a dose 2 or 3 times a day. I cannot emphasise enough that you should let the patient tell you, through his symptoms, what needs to be done. The less rigid and routine your prescribing the better the outcome will be.

Another rough guide is not to try more than approximately 4 or 6 different remedies without success before seeking more expert Homoeopathic advice. Obviously this will vary with the circumstances of each case and the experience of the prescriber. This is not a guide as to when to call on expert medical advice which should always be determined by the condition of the patient and carried out at whatever stage you would normally call upon such help whether or not you are treating them with Homoeopathic remedies. **Homoeopathic treatment, as described here, should always be an addition to whatever advice you would normally seek. It is never a substitute for calling your medical practitioner.**

When treating illness in children there are two very good signs that you have hit on the correct remedy: firstly, if the child vomits shortly after having the remedy, assuming he was not already vomiting all the time! You should not worry if part of the pill comes out as well, just wait and watch the child's condition. The second is if the child goes off to sleep. Do not disturb this sleep unless there are other indications that the child is not sleeping a peaceful, healing sleep. This sleep can be quite prolonged; my own son, when he was three, awoke screaming in the early hours one night with a very high fever and typical picture of *Belladonna*. He took the remedy and within ten minutes was fast asleep again. At 4 pm the following afternoon he awoke and came downstairs asking for breakfast!

It should now be clear that you need to monitor the patient in order to know what to do.

After subsequent doses of the selected remedy

Again several possibilities exist:

1. The patient improves after each dose and gradually needs the remedy less and less frequently until he is better. Nothing more can be added to this!

2. The patient gets better after each dose but requires it more and more frequently in order to sustain the benefit. This may well indicate the need for the next higher potency of that same remedy. If you don't have one then try plussing (see page 21). If this fails to hold the situation then review the case and see if there have been any changes or new information come to light that would enable you to select a more similar remedy which could carry on the work of the first remedy.

3. The patient improved at first but is now slipping back and a different set of symptoms has appeared. Your first prescription was right but a new remedy

is now needed. Base your selection on the new symptoms that have appeared. They will be a reliable guide to the second prescription.

4. There was initial improvement but now there is no response to the remedy and the same symptoms are still present. This probably means that the remedy was close but not quite close enough to give any sustained relief. You should reassess the case and choose another remedy, though it may first be worth trying a dose of the same remedy in a higher potency if you have it.

One further thing that will help you to be a successful prescriber; the more you enjoy it the easier it will be. Homoeopathy can be very satisfying if you do not get worried or weighed down by the 'burden' of finding a remedy. Keep it light and sometimes when things are not as clear as you would like them to be just trust and give the remedy you judge to be nearest. You can only do as well as your knowledge and experience allow which is just the same as the rest of us. Do not set your goals too high or else you will always be failing and there is nothing more demoralising. Homoeopathy is very safe and forgiving especially to honest beginners. Even a prescription of the wrong remedy can sometimes affect the picture of symptoms so as to make the right remedy more obvious and easily discerned.

May I wish you every success and satisfaction in your prescribing.

PART 2

Remedy Pictures
and Tables

**The suggestions for when to seek advice in the following sections
are only intended to be guidelines to help you decide when you need to
call on the expert help of your health care practitioner. Clearly your
own knowledge, experience and circumstances will all play a part in
your decision. The following guides do not aim to be totally
comprehensive. Complete books have been written on this subject
which will give much more information about when a condition is
likely to be serious or not. For this reason the guidelines here tend to
err on the cautious side.**

§3 Fevers

Remedy	Aconite	Sulphur	Arnica	Belladonna
Cause & onset	**Dry cold wind**, wet feet; exertion; anger; sudden fear or fright. **Rapid & violent** onset; evening, night.	Relapse after partial recovery or lingering symptoms; slower than *Bell.* or *Acon.*	Overexertion.	Cold; sunstroke; mental exertion. **Rapid onset, intense**.
Sensations	**Burning heat**. Mentally alert but frightened; senses very acute; tingling & numbness; like ice-water in the nerves. **Dryness** with extreme **thirst** for cold drinks; usually chill then heat then sweat; chilliness with internal heat < uncovering; shivering attacks.	**Burning** pains & discharges; internal heat, **flashes of heat** with sweat & chilliness; usually desire to uncover but may be chilly from it; chilliness from cold drinks; **thirst** for warm drinks; chill usually present, then dry heat, then sweat; sensitive to draughts, open air, odours; 11 am hunger. Insidious, continued or relapsing fevers.	Continued fevers; intense heat; dry heat; often sudden congestive chills, may be chilly uncovering; **great thirst** only **during the chill**.	**Intense burning heat; very high fever**, heat lingers on the hand; **severe pains, throbbings**; very **sensitive** to touch, light, jar or noise. Copious **thirst** with the heat, often for lemonade; may be thirsles; usually chill then heat & sweat; chilliness & **dry burning heat** may alternate. Tingling with numbness.
Modalities	< 12 pm evening, night; **light**; rising up; jar; touch; heat; covering.	< 12 am, 12 pm or daytime; **heat**; washing; changeable weather.	< **Touch**; motion; jar.	< 3 pm, 12 pm; **jar; motion; cold**; draught; touch; light; noise; rising; uncovering (& averse to); letting affected part hang down.
	> Perspiration; often uncovering.	> Warm drinks; open air.		> Still; lying down, on abdomen.
Concomitants	**Dry skin**, mouth, cough, heat. **Bounding pulse, hot congested head** & cold body. Flushed face alternates with paleness. Copious perspiration, on covered surfaces brings relief. Contracted pupils; stomach pains < cold drinks; scanty urine from fear.	**Perspiration at night with heat**, copious, mostly on upper part of the body; dry & red lips & mouth. Itching skin < heat; offensive acrid discharges. Oppression, burning, stitches in the chest; hot vertex of head with cold feet; soles of feet may burn at night.	Hot head or upper parts & cold extremities; perspiration can be absent. **Dusky spots on the skin** like bruises; mottled skin; coldness of parts lain on; catarrhs.	**Dry heat**, mouth & skin; **perspiration absent** usually, can be hot & steamy, < evening or night; sweat on covered parts only. **Bright red flushed skin**, later dusky; **hot congested head, cold limbs**; dilated pupils; **pulsations & dilated blood vessels; throbbings**. All in the head; tonsils, teeth, head or earache.
Peculiars	Sensations of crawling in the spine after a chill.	One sided symptoms. Left side.	One sided symptoms.	One sided symptoms. Right side.
Mentals and Generals (see texts)	**Intense, sudden**. Use **early in a fever**; if it lingers it is not *Aconite*. Acute panicky fear & restlessness. Hyperventilation maybe. Pains drive to despair. Many fears. Kicks off the covers.	Invigorated by cold open air. Not a very emotionally sensitive person; impatient & hurried; disorganised & messy; feels lethargic if he oversleeps. These **mentals may not be present** in fevers. Drowsy by day, restless by night, starts in sleep.	Delirium & stupor; **averse to being touched, so sore & bruised** all over, child screams out; bed feels hard causing restlessness. Morose wants to be left alone, not talked to. Prostrated; full of fears & nightmares; may say he is not sick when plainly is.	**Sudden & violent**. Usually **dull stupor**; can have **furious delirium; starting, twitching & jerking**; nervous excitability. **Swellings**. There is **no continued fever** in *Bell*. (see *Calc*.)

Fevers

Remedy	Calcarea	Mercurius	Apis	Natrum mur.
Cause & onset	Exertion; getting cold & wet.	Exertion	Fright; rage; jealousy; disappointment. **Rapid** onset.	Emotion; loss; grief; rejection; anger. Onset often at night.
Sensations	**Continued fever**, alternates with shivering; heat & chill alternate; internal heat & external coldness, < uncovering; heat with burning in blood vessels; photophobia; chill with thirst which can < the chill; dry heat.	**Chilliness**; creeping chilliness often in the evening & into the night; may alternate with flashes of heat; **violently sensitive to draughts. Metallic, sweet or foul taste**; not usually much thirst. Continued fever alternates with shivering; heat then chill.	**Intense burning heat**; continued fevers, stupor; **hot dry skin**, may alternate with sweats; chill, heat, sweat; chilliness < motion, may be < uncovering. **Thirstless** usually or for ice cold drinks or milk. **Stinging**; skin may be sensitive to touch, with tingling & numbness.	**Intense congestive heat; stupor or sleep**; internal heat with burning in blood vessels. **Dry** mouth & skin; thirst for **cold drinks during the chill** even; chilliness, teeth chatter, not relieved by warm wraps; chill heat sweat; chill may start in the extremities; **chill at 10–11 am.**
Modalities	< **Cold**; exertion; warm covers in the heat sometimes.	< **Night, heat, cold, sweat,** draught, uncovering, lying on right side, **everything!** > Lying, even temperature.	< 3–5 pm, **heat any form,** touch, pressure, after sleep. > **Cold**, open air, washing, motion.	< 10–11 am, eating, noise, music, heat in fever. > Sweat.
Concomitants	**Easy perspiration; hot congested head, cold feet**; may be cold on the scalp or in spots or areas only. **Swollen glands; sour odours; dilated pupils.**	**Copious salivation,** may drool yet feels dry & thirsty; **perspiration heavy & offensive,** often < them; night sweats. Cold extremities. **Offensiveness** -breath, sweat, discharges; foul mouth; enlarged **lymph nodes; catarrhs;** marked inflammations of skin, mouth; with pus or ulcers.	**Hot dry skin; perspiration often absent** or partial & **dries in between. Desires to uncover,** but may cause shivering. **Scanty urine; swelling & oedema;** inflammations look puffy & water filled. Tightness in abdomen with fear something will burst.	**Dry** mouth, lips & skin. **Perspiration** > everything except, sometimes, the headache. **Bursting headache with fever** & flushed face; chill may start in the limbs which go blue then on comes a headache. **Cold sore** on lips; **clear mucus** discharges, watery or like egg white.
Peculiars	Burning in blood vessels.	Metallic taste.	Right side or right to left.	Desires cold drinks in the chill; burning in blood vessels.
Mentals and Generals (see texts)	Often chilly people full of congestions & weakness; < exertion; may be of relaxed & flabby build. Often follows *Bell.* if the fever becomes continuous.	Unhealthy appearance; trembling, weak, tires easily; delirium; dull mind or agitation & restlessness leading to hurry & impulsiveness, even driven out of bed at night. Colds go to chest.	**Apathetic, wingeing, weepy; irritable;** even suspicious or jealous; stupor in heat. Awkwardness, clumsy; says he is not sick. **Undeveloped or suppressed rashes.** *Puls.* may follow it.	Periodicity. There may be intense fever with delirium & constant talking.

Fevers

Remedy	Arsenicum	Pulsatilla	Bryonia	Gelsemium
Cause & onset	Exertion; heat; flu that lingers.	Getting feet wet; flu that lingers.	Exposure to cold, especially if sweating; hurt feelings. **Slow** onset; mornings.	Emotions, fear, shock, anticipation, bad news; mild winters & weather; lingering flu. **Slow** onset, pm or night.
Sensations	**Burning heat** > heat. **Burning pains** > heat. Burning or ice in blood vessels; **continued** fever with **stupor, delirium**. Intense **shivering**, alternates with heat. Chill, dry heat, sweat. Irregular chills, heat, sweats. Aching bones in chill; **thirst** for hot drinks in chill, for **sips in the heat & copious for cold** in the sweat.	**Burning heat**; continued fever, very hot at night; dry heat. **Alternations** – heat, chilly, sweats, shivering. Chill at 4 pm; in spots; often starts in hands & feet with pains in the limbs; flitting chilliness; **wandering pains**. **Thirstless** in fever with a dry foul mouth; may be thirsty before chill.	**Burning heat; continued fever**; high fever, stupor, delirium. **Dry heat, mouth; intense thirst** for large quantities of **cold** drinks at long intervals; burning internally, in blood vessels; chilliness with internal heat; chill, heat, sweat; usually wants to uncover. Pains flit here & there.	**Burning heat. Stupor, dazed**, talks as if delirious; continued fever; heat prickles over the body; **chills run up & down the spine;** chill, heat, sweat; chill may be absent or alternate. **Numbness & disturbed sensations. Thirstless** or little. In flu that lingers – chilly & heat, not ill, not well, weak & heavy.
Modalities	< **Night**, 1–2 am, **cold** except head, draughts, uncovering, motion, exertion. > **Heat** except head, company.	< **Evening**, night, **heat in any form, close room**, 4 pm chill, fatty or rich foods, cough by lying. > **Cool, open air, gentle motion**, washing, lying on painful side, cough by sitting.	< 9 pm, evening, night, **motion**, jar, **heat, sun**, rising up, noise, after eating. > **Firm pressure, still, cold, open air**, perspiration.	< Afternoon, 10 am & worsens through the day, lying with the head low. > **Stimulants** – alcohol, coffee, etc., lying propped up, sweating, urinating.
Concomitants	Dry heat; Perspiration with copious **thirst** for **cold** drinks which > fever & pains, followed by great **exhaustion**; prolonged sweat; external **coldness**, icy coldness. Catarrhs; excoriating discharges.	**Dry** heat, lips; **hot** head, distended vessels; **desire to uncover, for fresh air. Thick, bland, yellow/green discharges;** often some form of **stomach upset**; coated tongue. Perspiration may be profuse or one sided; profuse morning sweat.	Generalised bodily soreness; joint pains, lies quite still; right sided pains > lying on painful side. **Headache** is usual, > still & pressure. **Dryness**, heat, lips, mouth; white tongue; constipation, large, hard & dry stools. Perspiration > all complaints. Eyes sore. Painful distension after eating.	**Dusky, red, congested face.** Ptosis; physically **so weak**. Hot head & back, cold extremities; stiff achy neck & back; bursting **congestive** headache from neck or **occiput to forehead & eyes**; eyes sore. Incontinence from paralysis of sphincters. Coryza.
Peculiars	Red hot needle pains; burning or ice in blood vessels.	**One sidedness** – chill, heat or sweat.	One sided. Burning in blood vessels.	Headache > copious urination.
Mentals and Generals (see texts)	Great **restlessness; anxiety; fear; prostration**; disproportionate **weakness; chilly**; desires **company**, fears being alone. Possessive & fastidious.	Gentle, mild, **clingy, weepy, cuddly** children; **changeability**; nervous & fidgety; may be irritable. Palpitation with anxiety, must uncover. Often looks well even when is not.	Much < **motion** in any form. **Extreme irritability**, does not wish to be disturbed, talked to, or to move. Mentally dull & may be homesick. Dizzy in warm rooms; sleepless if stuffy.	**Feeling of great weight & tiredness.** Drowsy, weak, dull & indifferent. Wants to be left alone because is **too tired** to talk or be irritable. So weak & heavy he just lies still; **slow, congestive complaints**. Trembling, paresis, clumsy, uncoordinated.

Fevers

Remedy	Ferrum phos.	Rhus tox.	Phosphorus	Eupator. perf.
Cause & onset	Overexertion. **Slower** than *Bell*.	**Overexertion**; cold & damp; suppressed sweat. Onset especially at night.	Electrical changes in the weather; mental exertions. Onset often at night.	
Sensations	Dry heat; not so intense as *Bell*. More **alert**, they take notice of what goes on arround them; can be dull as they tire. Chill at 4 pm, may be absent; thirst during fever. Numbness of parts of the body.	**Dry burning heat**; high fever; continued. Mild, persistent delirium with laborious dreams; muttering. Intense heat, **restless & dry tongue** with it. **Sore & bruised** aches. Usually chilly, **averse to uncovering**, shivers on least exposure. Chill may be absent, heat, sweat; cold in single parts with internal heat, sweat cold in single parts with internal heat. **Thirst** for cold drinks or milk, may < though.	**Dry burning heat. Burning pains.** Sensation of intense heat running up the back. **Unquenchable thirst for cold drinks in burning heat which** >. Vomits warm drinks. **Senses are over sensitive** to all impressions – noise, light, odour, touch. More alert often; continued fever, stupor, delirium.	Burns all over with heat but feels hotter to touch than the temperature justifies; **chills especially at 7–9 am**, in the back; **great thirst for ice cold** which < stomach & shivering. Violent headache with the chill; chill, heat, little sweat usually.
Modalities	< **Cold**, open air, uncovering, exertion, standing, noise, sour food. > Gentle motion.	< **Evening, night. Cold, damp, first motion** – aches, during sleep, rest, overexertion. > **Heat, continued motion** – aches, pressure, rubbing, sweat.	< Evening, lying on painful side. > Cold drinks, cold food, rubbing, sleep, walking in open air.	< **Motion**, sweat can < headache.
Concomitants	**Hot head, cold extremities; hot & flushed; circular red patches on cheeks; flushes & pales easily**; surgings of blood. Dry lips; profuse **perspiration** that weakens. Tendency to bleed; blood discharges; **epistaxis** with fever or headache. Bodily soreness, back ache.	**Joints, tendons & ligaments swollen stiff & painful.** Dry mouth, dry sore throat; **cold sore on lips**; sweat may be profuse; sweat with heat & shivering, may > the severe aching in the bones (*Eup.*). Back ache > lying on something hard. Itchy skin eruptions & inflammations.	Dry heat, mouth; perspiration with the heat. **Easy bleeding.** Restless & fidgety, later weak & prostrated.	**Severe aching pains in bones as if they would break** leads to this remedy. Perspiration absent or scanty with the heat. Congestive, bursting headache, dare not move for the pain; flushed face. Sudden coryza with sneezing & red eyes before the aches; eyeballs sore (*Bry. Gels.*); dry hacking cough; stomach upset; may vomit bile.
Peculiars	One sided; right side.	**Triangular red tip** to tongue. Sensation of heat in blood vessels.	One sided; left side.	Bilious vomiting between chill & heat.
Mentals and Generals (see texts)	**Flushed, tired & easily exhausted; bleeding.** Less restless than *Acon.*, less violent than *Bell*. Often used early in a fever when no other remedy is clearly indicated, when there are no clear distinguishing features.	**Pains > motion, restless, anxious**; sleepless & irritable; fearful < night. **Feels bruised & sore, aching, tearing pains < cold.** Stiff, lame & bruised on first motion then eased but tires & rests when becomes stiff & restless again.	**Restless, overexcited state leading to weakness & exhaustion.** Startles easily; may have lots of fears; delicate people, they like company & often sleep on the right side. Rarely used early in an acute illness.	Similar to *Bryonia* & *Phos*. **Marked aching in all bones** with **soreness of flesh.** Dare not move for the pain **though** the pains may make him restless.

Fevers

Remedy	Spongia	Hepar sulph.	Nux vomica	Pyrogen
Cause & onset	Exertion. **Slower onset;** pm & evening often.	Cold dry winds.	Overindulgence; stimulants (coffee, alcohol etc.); mental overexertion. Cold dry winds.	
Sensations	**Dryness;** roughness & **dryness** of mucous membranes; burning heat with external coldness; chill, heat, sweat.	**Marked chilliness from slightest exposure, uncovering, even of single parts. Hypersensitive** to touch, pain, cold; **splinter like pains; pains** < **cold.** Burning heat; intense; continued fever; delirium; thirst with the heat; chill, heat, sweat.	**Extreme chilliness from slightest exposure or uncovering** like *Hepar.*; < slightest **movement, drinking; waves of chills,** often begin in the extremities or back. Short dry heat followed by intense heat with hot sweats; stupor; delirium; sometimes thirsty but may cause bloating.	**Fever full of violent pulsations & intense restlessness.** Chilliness that no fire can warm (*Nux v., Gels.*); creeping chills in back with thumping heart; little chills & little shiverings throughout the body. Sore & bruised, bed feels hard (*Arn.*).
Modalities	< Lying down.	< Morning & evening, **cold,** pressure, motion, exertion. > Heat, wet weather	< Morning, **dry cold, open air,** uncovering, noise, motion, rich stimulant foods. > Evening, sleep, sitting, in bed.	< Beginning to move.
Concomitants	Raw sore throat with larynx sensitive to touch like *Phos.* Croup. Perspiration absent.	**Offensive odours, sour or cheesy discharges,** profuse, thick; suppurating tendency – boils, ulcers; catarrhs; croup. Dry heat with sweaty hands when put out of bed; perspires easily with the heat; perspires all night without relief.	**Very red face;** dry heat or perspiration with the heat. **Often associated with an upset stomach.** In chills hands are cold & purple.	**Temperature & pulse out of phase** – high temperature with low pulse & vice versa. Pulse may be **very** rapid. Bursting headache with intense restlessness; bed feels hard because of sore bruised sensation. Copious urination of clear water with the fever.
Peculiars				Temperature & pulse out of normal relationship.
Mentals and Generals (see texts)	**Anxiety, fear** of death, of suffocation, with palpitations & uneasiness in the heart region. Similar to *Aconite* but it lacks the febrile excitement. A fullness in the chest too; wakens with great fear.	**Irritable & hypersensitive; intense suffering out of proportion;** faints with the pain. Delicate sensitive people; discontented & nothing pleases them; cross & pick quarrels; sudden violent impulses.	**Oversensitive, irritable & touchy;** imagines offences, critical, hurried, intolerant, impulsive, impatient. May keep all this controlled & not show it.	

Fevers (See also *Dulcamara* and *Euphrasia* for further possibilities)

Baptisia	China	Coffea	Hyoscyamus	Merc. cyan.
Rapid onset.	**In flu that lingers.**			Rapid onset. Night.
High fever. **Sudden septic states. Feels stupid at first & rapidly prostrated.**	**Continued debility with chilliness**. Sensitive to touch, motion & cold air. Thirst before the chill comes on; great thirst in the sweat.	Dry heat at night with delirium. Intense heat, **Chilliness** in back with dry heat in bed; shivering, external heat; feeling of heat in bed yet averse to uncovering; chilly in the evening or night; chill, heat, sweat.	**Continued fever**; very high fever; **stupor, complete stupor**; delirium, jerkings; dry heat, burning heat with sleeplessness; alternating chill & heat; chill then sweat; burning in blood vessels.	**Icy coldness**; great sensitivity to cold; very cold extremities. **Rawness & soreness.**
	< Night, alternate days, touch, motion, cold air, loss of vital fluids.	< Warm covering.	> In bed.	< Evening.
Dull red face, drugged, besotted appearance; red, dusky, comatose; drops asleep while answering questions. **Foul mouth** & throat; discharges very **offensive**; sour perspiration. Solids gag but fluids go down all right.	Weariness of limbs with desire to stretch, move or change position.		Perspiration absent; distended blood vessels; warm pale skin.	**Coldness**; skin cold & moist; **trembling; putridity & ulceration.** Complaints of mouth, throat & pharynx; **follicular tonsilitis** with a thick white coating on the tonsils; ulcerations & rawness.
Dissociation of parts – feels scattered & cannot get himself together (*Pyr.*).			Burning in blood vessels.	
Sinks rapidly into a stupid, stuporose state; **great prostration.**	Anaemic, pallid, weak.	Always ready to weep.		**Early, rapid & extreme prostration.**

Fevers: When to seek advice

Urgently, Right now!

- If the fever is very high – approximately 106°F (41.1°C) or above, in any patient.
- For any fever in the young infant – less than 4 months. The very young can stop feeding and rapidly become very ill. The more lethargic, weak and ill the infant, the greater is the urgency and need for expert advice. If necessary you should be prepared to take your child to your health practitioner's surgery or even to hospital. Do whatever is necessary to get a very sick young infant seen.
- If the conscious level of the patient is affected – drowsiness, confusion, lethargy and unresponsiveness.
- If there are fits or convulsions.
- If the neck becomes stiff.
- If the breathing is very rapid or laboured.
- Look at the whole patient and ask yourself the question 'How sick?' If the answer is 'Very' then seek advice, even if none of the above categories apply. With a young child the mother will often just know something is seriously wrong and she should trust this knowledge and act accordingly.

Within 24 hours

- If the fever is persistently above about 104°F (40°C) and will not respond to the following measures:
  1. Homoeopathic treatment.
  2. Open a window and keep the room cool but not cold.
  3. Cover with only one blanket.
  4. **Tepid** sponge the whole body. Do not use cold water.
- For fevers in children of 4–6 months and persistent fevers in older children. As a rough guide, if a fever persists more than a day or two in a child under 2 years then consider seeking advice. The older the child the longer you can wait so long as there are no other signs of serious illness.

  Remember to give plenty of clear fluids – water and fruit juices. Breastfeeding infants will require more frequent feeds and may take water and fruit juice in addition. Solid food is not necessary for anyone with an acute fever and will usually be rejected anyway. (See the section on diarrhoea and vomiting.)

Refer to other chapters as necessary.

§4 Headaches

Remedy	Belladonna	Natrum mur.	Arsenicum	Sulphur
Cause & onset	Exposure of the head to cold, even a haircut. Suppressed coryza. **Sudden & violent onset.**	Grief, humiliation, eyestrain. Onset on waking, 10–11 am.	Exertion, excitement, getting heated. Onset often 1–3 pm.	Missed meals.
Site		Right eye especially. Occiput extending down the spine.	**Forehead and occiput.**	
Sensations	**Pulsating, bursting,** hammering pains. **Burning,** tearing, shooting, stabbing pains. Sensation as if the brain was going up & down. A heavy head. So severe he may roll the head despite > motion.	Dreadful **bursting, pressing, throbbing,** hammering, as if in a vice, crushing. **Periodical.** Must go to bed & be perfectly quiet.	Sick, severe headaches. **Throbbing & burning, waves of pain.** Congestion, brain feels loose. **Periodicity, very chilly; wraps up** but wants the head cool. Neuralgic pains need warmth though.	Sick headache. **Throbbing,** pressing, **burning. Heat in the vertex > cold.** Periodical, every 7 days. Head is sensitive. Burning in the palms & soles. Heaviness in the head. Constricting sensation.
Modalities	< Jar, motion, stepping, touch, cold & draft, uncovering, light, rising up, bending head forwards, stooping, noise, lying. > Pressure on head, drawing head back.	< 10–11 am, noise. > Sleep, sweating.	Congestion < **heat,** light, motion, jar, noise, 1–2 am. > Cold, cold air or water, lying down in a dark room.	< **12 am & 12 pm,** stooping, jar, light, after eating, cold drinks, motion. > Warm room & applications, hot drinks, head uncovered.
Head & Face	**Congestion, hot head. Redness & swelling.**		**Congestion. Hot head.** Head in constant motion sometimes.	**Marked congestion.** Red engorged face.
Concomitants	Dizziness on moving the head, < stooping. Dilated pupils. Rush of blood to the head.	Zigzag lines & flickering lights may come before the headache. **Dryness of mucous membranes.**	Usually has nausea & vomiting. Fever headaches.	Nausea & vomiting of bile. Red eyes with tearing, red face. Flickering lights before headaches.
Peculiar		Crack in the middle of the lower lip.		
Mentals and Generals (see texts)	Jerking & twitching.	May be weepy but does not let others see it. Anger from isolation.	Generally chilly & > heat but head is > cold. **Anxiety, restlessness, prostration, pallor.**	Feels dull and stupid. Hungry at 11 am. Itchy skin < heat. Hates standing.

Headaches

Remedy	Nux vomica	Pulsatilla	Ferrum phos.	Gelsemium
Cause & onset	Stimulants, overexertion, night watching, sweating.	Overeating, icecream, before menses.		Cold, fear, embarrassment. Slow onset.
Site		One sided. Often sides & temples.	Forehead to occiput, especially right side. Vertex, sides.	Especially occipital.
Sensations	Tension pains especially drawing. Piercing, sticking, tearing, burning stinging. Neuralgic pains. Faints with the pain & weeps. Sensation of a great weight on the vertex.	Throbbing, constricting, congestive headaches. Periodical. Thirstless.	Blinding, catarrhal, bursting, hammering, pressing, boring pains. Stitching. Vertex sensitive to cold. Head feels cold or hot.	Hammering, pulsating, congestive pains. Neuralgic headache in temples, over eyes, with nausea & vomiting.
Modalities	< Heat, after eating, rising, open air, moving eyes. > Perfect quiet, covered up.	< Heat, lying & sitting quiet. Motion of eyes, stooping. > Cold, cold applications, fresh air etc. Slow motion in open air, pressure, menses.	< Wrapping up, motion, jar, stepping, coughing, light, noise. > Cold air or applications. Lying down (is often compelled to), pressure.	< Motion (it is impossible, so tired, can't stand up). Neuralgia < vomiting. > Lying in bed propped up by pillows & quite still, passing copious urine, sweating.
Head & Face		Hot head.	Flushes of heat & a red face may alternate with paleness. Head hot & full. Feet cold.	Congested. Face flushed & dusky. Eyes glazed, pupils dilated.
Concomitants	Backache < lying down, must get up & walk. Pain with nausea and sour vomiting. Easy perspiration & least chill or draft causes headache with coryza.	Sour food causes vomiting. With menses or suppressed menses.	Dizziness, coryza, vomiting or sore scalp.	With gastroenteritis, scanty urine, nausea, trembling, eyes glassy, cold extremities.
Peculiars			Hot, full head; frontal headache > nosebleed.	
Mentals and Generals (see texts)	Chilly person & > heat except head. With stomach or liver troubles; with piles. Irritable, oversensitive, touchy.	Weepy, clingy & changeable.	Dark circles under the eyes; sallow look; circumscribed redness on the cheeks.	Profound exhaustion; great tiredness & weakness; heavy limbs.

Headaches

Remedy	Bryonia	Lachesis	Lycopodium	Spigelia
Cause & onset	**Cold**; washing in cold water when sweating. **Slow onset.**	**On waking.** From sun, springtime.	Taking cold; hunger; suppressed catarrh.	Taking cold; sun headaches. Onset at sunrise.
Site	Forehead & occiput.	**Left side or left to right.**		**Occiput to above eyes, especially left** eye which waters.
Sensations	**Bursting pressure pain > pressure, as if the skull would split open.** Fullness & heaviness. Throbbing on motion. Sharp pains stabbing over the eyes. Wakes with a congested headache. **Thirsty & dry.**	**Bursting, pulsating pains. Sensation of weight & pressure.** Pressure & burning on the vertex. Throbbing **waves of pain.** Senses are oversensitive. Congested pains. Sleeps into a headache.	**Throbbing, pressing, bursting pains. Hot head,** wants it uncovered; cold extremities.	**Intense pains; shooting, burning, pulsating, tearing, stabbing & stitching. Neuralgic pains.** Pain on moving the eyes, intolerable. From sunrise & worsens until noon & declines until sunset.
Modalities	< **Slightest motion,** any exertion. **Warm & stuffy room.** Sitting up, light, after eating, coughing. > **Lying still in a dark room.** Neuralgia may be > heat.	< **Entering sleep, on waking,** touch, heat, noise. > **Firm pressure,** the onset of a discharge.	< 4–8 pm; **heat;** warm wraps; lying down; noise. > **Cool air;** motion; return of a thick yellow nasal discharge.	< **Daytime; motion** – even mental exertion; eating; noise; warmth; cold, damp, rainy days; eyes < touch. > Lying with head high; rest; dry air.
Head & Face	Hot head. Somewhat besotted, mottled, purple.	**Congested head.** Mottled purple face. Pale face sometimes.		
Concomitants	Headache **with every acute illness.** Red congested eyes, soreness in eyeballs. Often nosebleed with the headache.	Dizziness, nausea & vomiting. Weak pulse. Dim vision, flickering, loss of sight.	Hunger with headache.	**Vertigo, dizzy** from looking down. Palpitations. Stiff neck & shoulders > warmth.
Peculiars	Nausea & faintness on rising.			Eyes feel too large with the pain, intolerable.
Mentals & Generals (see texts)	**Bruised feeling all over; irritable.** Must keep perfectly **still**; dull mind, slow, sluggish, passive. Headache often precedes other complaints.	Cannot stand the touch of clothes on the skin; loquacity.	A chilly person but wants cool air for the head. Nervous excitement & prostration.	

Headaches

(See also *Aconite, Allium cepa, Calcarea, Eupator. perf., Euphrasia, Ipecacuanha, Kali bich., Kali carb., Mercurius, Phosphorous, Rhus tox., Silica* and *Spongia* for further possibilities)

Remedy	Iris	Sanguinaria		
Cause & onset	After relaxing from a mental stress.	Sun; overeating rich food or wine.		
Site	Frontal; right temple.	**Occiput to above right eye** or temple; **right** sided.		
Sensations	**Sick headaches.** Usually begin with a **blur before the eyes.** Burning from tongue down to stomach with nausea & vomiting. Periodicity every 4 or 6 weeks. Scalp feels constricted.	Sick headaches; sun headaches. Feels head must burst; eyes as if being pressed out. Palms & soles hot, burning. Congestive hot bursting headache. Periodicity, every 7th or 3rd day.		
Modalities	< Rest.	< Daytime, rises & falls with the sun; light; motion; noise; night.		
Head & Face				
Concomitants	**Nausea & sour vomiting.** Profuse secretions of ropy saliva. Watery stools burn the anus.	Nausea & vomiting, bilious vomiting; faintness, all gone feeling but not a hunger; chills; burning palms & soles; circumscribed redness of the cheeks.		
Peculiars				
Mentals and Generals (see texts)				

Headaches: When to seek advice

Urgently, Right now!

- If the level of consciousness is affected – drowsiness, confusion, etc.
- For any severe unexpected headache.
- If there is stiffness of the neck and/or high fever (above approximately 104°F, 40°C) and/or photophobia.
- If the headache follows a head injury, especially if there is drowsiness or vomiting. (See the first aid section.)

Within 24 hours

- For headaches with any symptoms involving other parts of the nervous system, such as disturbances of sensation, especially vision and dizziness or any disturbed capacity to initiate movement, such as speech difficulty or weakness.
- If the headache is continuous with no signs of improvement over several days even if the headache is mild.

§5 Eye complaints

Remedy	Aconite	Belladonna	Apis	Pulsatilla
Cause & onset	**Cold**, especially **dry cold winds.** **Sudden & violent.**	**Cold.** **Sudden onset.**	Emotional stress, jealousy, anger. **Rapid onset.**	
Side		Right.	Right to left.	
Sensations & appearance	**Violent aching, burning. Congested; marked & rapid swelling;** bright red.	**Intense burning heat; dryness; throbbing. Bright red or dusky later; swelling.**	**Burning & stinging pains; inflammations;** congested blood vessels; photophobia; iritis. **Swelling, oedema** of the lids, of the conjunctiva.	Sore & itching; lids. **Thirstless** with a dry mouth. Follicular conjunctivitis.
Modalities	< **Light.**	< 3 pm & night, **motion, jar, light,** pressure, cold. > Still.	< **Heat** in any form. > **Cold** in any form, washing.	< **Heat** in any form. > Washing in **cold or tepid water,** gentle motion.
Discharges	**None** or a little watery mucus only; **never thick or purulent.**	**No pus.**	Profuse tears.	**Thick, profuse, yellow/ green, bland discharge.**
Concomitants	Contracted pupils; dry & thirsty.	Hot head, cold feet; dryness, may be very thirsty, often thirstless.	Any rash, often dry & rough; scanty urine maybe.	
Peculiars			Swelling may come & go rapidly.	
Mentals and Generals (see texts)	Restlessness, anxiety, fear; nervous excitement, violence, etc.	Not a prolonged lingering state; short & sharp.		Colds go to the eyes; recurrent styes. A clingy, whiny, weepy child; desires fresh air.

Eye complaints

Remedy	Argentum nit.	Sulphur	Mercurius	Rhus tox.
Cause & onset		Colds.	Colds.	Cold damp wind; suppressed sweat.
Side				
Sensations & appearance	**Photophobia. Swelling & redness;** swelling of lids, of conjunctiva; ulceration.	**Burning heat.** Red & sore round eyes; ulceration of lids.	**Photophobia; burning & tearing pains;** fog or mist before the eyes. Inflammation of lids, of conjunctiva; **swelling;** eyes spasmodically closed; ulceration.	**Bruised sore pains;** photophobia; iritis. **Swelling,** eyes closed from it, or lids, of conjunctiva; red lids.
Modalities	< **Warm room.** > **Cold applications.**	< 12 am or pm. **Washing or bathing eye,** heat.	< Night. **Heat, cold,** draught, sweat.	< Morning, **cold,** moving eyeball. > **Heat.**
Discharges	Profuse, purulent discharge.	Mucus & pus.	**Copious acrid tears; green or yellow discharge; offensive.**	Copious, purulent, mucous discharge; sticky lids in morning.
Concomitants		Itching of skin < heat; facial eruptions.	Enlarged glands; offensiveness, foul mouth with flabby tongue & spongy gums; copious salivation.	Rashes, especially if vesicular
Peculiars			Metallic taste.	
Mentals and Generals (see texts)	Desires cold, open air.	Every cold settles in the eyes.	Every cold settles in the eyes.	Rheumatic joints; restlessness & fever.

Eye complaints

(See also *Allium cepa* and *Natrum mur.* for further possibilities)

Silica	Euphrasia	Arsenicum	Bryonia	Hepar sulph.
Cold damp weather. Trauma or foreign bodies.			Cold; cold dry winds; suppressing a sweat.	**Cold dry winds.**
Photophobia; burning & stinging. Suppuration of the lid margins; eyes inflamed from trauma or a foreign body (after its removal).	Cutting pains extending into the head; pressure as if by sand in eyes; dryness; burning, biting, violent itching – must rub. **Swelling** of conjunctiva & lids, red inflamed & sore.	**Burning.** Swelling may occur, bag like under the eyes with oedema; ulceration.	Stiching, burning & smarting; pressing pain; sore aching & **cannot bear to be touched.** Swollen lids; red conjunctiva; dilated veins.	**Oversensitive** to pains, touch & **air**; boring, sore pains.
	< Open air, windy weather, light.	< Cold washing or heat (burning).	< 9 pm often, **moving eyeballs**, heat, light. > Cold.	< **Cold & dry**, touch, pressure. > **Heat**, damp.
Thin, watery, copious discharge; thick, yellow, bloody discharge.	**Copious acrid watery discharge**; eye discharge may be purulent; a tendency to accumulate sticky mucus on cornea removed by blinking.	**Acrid.** Thin, bloody increasing to thick & bloody.	Watery.	Thick, purulent, offensive, cheesy discharge; bloody catarrhal discharge.
	Fluent bland coryza during a cold; < lying down at night. Throbbing, catarrhal headache; cough < daytime, > night.		**Headache**, commonly; coryza, sneezing. When joint complaints have gone to the eyes, iritis etc.	
		Burning > **heat.**		
	Chilly; chill, fever, sweat; fever mostly in the day.	**Restless, chilly, anxious,** miserable & weak out of proportion to the illness; thirsty for sips of ice cold water little & often.	**Thirsty,** dry, irritable & wants to be on his own, etc.	**Chilly, oversentive & irritable** patient.

Eyes: When to seek advice

Urgently, Right now!

- If there is any deterioration or loss of vision.
- If any eye pain is severe.
- If the eye is damaged by a foreign body or chemical. Wash out liquid irritants immediately, usually copious clean water is required, and seek advice without delay.

Within 24 hours

- If there is a thick yellow or green discharge flowing from the eye.
- If significant eye pain persists.
- If bright lights cause significant pain, especially if the eye is red mainly around the iris or the pupil is irregular and does not react normally to changes of light.
- If there is a rash, such as shingles, or an infection on the face close to or involving the eye in any way.

Refer to other chapters as necessary

§6 Ear complaints

Remedy	Aconite	Belladonna	Ferrum phos.	Pulsatilla
Cause & Onset	Cold; cold dry wind. **Sudden & violent.**	**Cold**; exposure of the head, even a hair cut; draught. **Sudden onset.**	Cold. Throat went to ear.	After rashes like measles, scarlet fever etc.
Side		**Right side.**		
Sensations	Intense, throbbing, cutting, stinging, burning, tearing pains; child screams with pain.	**Intense throbbing & burning pains.**	Deep drawing pain; stitching; itches; hears noises.	Pains with chilliness yet wants the open air. Deafness & noises; damage ever since infection. **Dryness without thirst**; bad taste in the morning.
Modalities	< **Noise** is intolerable, covering & a warm room.	< 3 pm, night, **jar**, motion, touch, cold. > Heat, stillness.	< Noise, exertion, open air, jar. > Gentle motion.	<**Evening, night, Heat,** rest. > Slow motion, lying on painful side.
Discharges	**No suppuration.** This remedy comes early in an infection.	No suppuration. This remedy comes early like *Aconite.*	**Suppuration**; purulent discharge.	**Thick, yellow/ green, bland, purulent discharge;** foetid; sometimes bloody.
Concomitants	**Fever; thirst & dryness;** congested face.	Bright **red; dry intense fever; high fever;** thirst & dryness but may be thirstless; hot head & cold feet.	Cold extremities or hot all over; eustachian catarrh; pain & swelling of parotid.	
Peculiars				
Mentals & Generals (see texts)	Must be carried. **Senses are hyperacute;** irritability; restlessness etc.	May be delirious, drowsy, jerking & starting, etc.	**Flushes easily or pale;** malaise, low fever; thirsty.	**Pitiful weeping, clingy, contrary & never satisfied; changeable** etc.

Ear complaints

Remedy	Silica	Sulphur	Mercurius	Chamomilla
Cause & Onset	Damp cold weather; suppressed sweat	Colds.	Cold & damp.	Air, wind; anger, temper. Evening often.
Side				
Sensations	Eustachian catarrh; deafness; hissing & roaring; hearing returns with a snap; may be chilly.	**Burning, stinging pains.** Strange noises; eventually deafness; congested head & wants fresh air.	**Stinging pains** like *Apis*; raw & burning; chronic ear infections.	**Sharp pains**; stitching; heat & fullness in ear; roaring & ringing.
Modalities		< 12 am & 12 pm, **washing, heat.**	< **Night, draught, heat & cold**, sweating.	< 9 am, 9 pm to 12 midnight, cold air (ears alone are very sensitive). > Heat, being carried.
Discharges	Offensive, thick, yellow discharge; offensive, watery, curdy discharge.	Copious, **offensive**, purulent, bloody discharge. Acrid & burning.	**Horribly stinking green discharge**; thick, acrid pus; bloody discharge.	
Concomitants	Sweat about upper part of body or head; offensive sweat.	Eruptions with itching < heat & water. Congested face.	**Offensive sweats, fevers, chills** especially creeping chills; thirsty with a moist, foul mouth, even salivation; flabby tongue & soft gums; swollen glands – parotid, lymph nodes in neck; stiff neck.	Often thirsty.
Peculiars			Metallic taste.	
Mentals and Generals (see texts)	May be needed to finish off after *Pulsatilla*.			Puts his hand to cover his ear; **fussy, irritable & angry, sensitive, mad, whining, never satisfied** but not cuddly like *Puls*. The emotional state often leads to this prescription.

Ear complaints (See also *Calcarea*, *Kali bich*. and *Natrum mur*. for further possibilities)

Hepar sulph.	Allium cepa	Lycopodium	Nux vomica	Lachesis
Dry cold wind. Quite sudden onset.	Cold damp & penetrating winds. Coryza to ears.	Cold; after scarlet fever.	Cold, especially cold dry weather.	
	Left to right.	Right or **Right to left.**		**Left or left to right.**
Sticking, tearing pains; bursting pain before it discharges; when pus has already formed.	Violent ache, drawing, stitching, tearing pains; jerking pains from throat to ears; pains in forehead to ears.	Tearing, bursting, pressing pains; deafness.	Stitches when swallowing; hypersensitive senses; itching in ear.	**Pulsations in the ear;** pain in the ear **with sore throat;** very **sensitive meatus** – violent spasmodic coughing or tickling in throat if anything touches inside the meatus.
< **Night, cold, draught, uncovering.** > **heat**, damp weather	< Warmth.	< 4–8 pm. > Cool air (the ear)	< Morning, **cold, least uncovering or draught,** noise, in bed.	< **On waking, after sleep or entering sleep, heat,** touch, pressure, constriction.
Yellow, thick with a cheesy odour; may be purulent & bloody.	Purulent.	Thick, yellow, offensive.		**A septic state with purulent discharge.**
May sweat without any >.	**Acrid watery coryza with bland watery eye discharge, both profuse.**	Dry cough; chilly; eczema & rashes around & behind the ears.	Often with a digestive upset; < eating.	With **sore throat** (see); neck sensitive to touch.
Hypersensitivity of nerves; chilly; oversensitive to **touch, pain & cold.** Screaming, biting, kicking child.		Especially in an emaciating, wrinkled child.	**Chilly, irritable, oversensitve & easily angered;** takes cold easily. See *Fevers* & *Nose*.	**Bluish, purplish inflammations.**

Ears: When to seek advice

Urgently, Right now!

- If there is also drowsiness, severe headache, stiffness of the neck or severe lethargy.

Within 24 hours

- If a baby persistently pulls or rubs an ear. Frequently this indicates an ear infection. Most mild ear infections will settle in time without any treatment, but their progress should be monitored and homoeopathic treatment will help them to settle quicker.
- If the earache is severe or if any earache accompanies measles.
- Any ear discharge.
- If the bony lump behind the ear (mastoid bone) becomes tender or red.
- If the hearing is significantly and persistently impaired.

Refer to other chapters as necessary.

§7 Nose & sinuses

Remedy	Pulsatilla	Kali bich.	Natrum mur.	Silica
Cause & onset	Getting wet.		10–11 am with sneezing.	Cold, damp; getting wet; suppressed sweat.
Site				
Sensations	**Loss of smell;** bad odour & taste; pain in the face through the nose; coryza with sneezing, stuffing up of the nose in the evening & copious flow in morning; nose stuffs up indoors & evenings.	Hard pain at **root of nose;** pulsating; very sore inside; dry sensation; **bones very sore;** shooting pains in the cheek bones. Dry sensation; dryness with pressure pain at root of nose.	Smarting pain in nose; loss of smell & taste; **dry mouth** & lips; sometimes bitter taste. Chill at 10–11 am.	Loss of smell & taste.
Modalities	< **Warm room, heat.** > **Open air** – nose discharges & clears, gentle motion.	< **Night, morning**, damp weather stooping, motion. > Warmth, pressure.	< Morning, 10–11 am till noon, exposure to fresh air. > Sweat.	> Cold, dry.
Discharges	**Bland, thick, yellow/green discharges.** Blocked nose or water discharge in the evening; copious discharge in the morning & nose clears.	**Copious, thick, viscid, stringy, yellow or white or green.** Jelly-like mucus. Foetid; offensive; in an acute illness may be acrid & watery. Dries up if exposed to cold & a headache begins.	**Copious watery or white like egg white;** excessive secretion; dry crusty; post nasal catarrh.	Hard crusts accumulate; horrible, foetid, bloody discharges; nosebleeds.
Concomitants	**Thirstless with a dry mouth;** coated tongue; lips chapped & peel; bleeding from nose.	Often begins with dim vision & then a violent headache; dizziness.	Cold sores on lips; watery eye discharges; sneezing spells; cough with bursting headache; hoarseness; cannot sleep in a warm room.	Crusty eruption at junction of mucous membranes & skin; rough lips, crack & peel.
Peculiars	**One sided** complaints.	**Stringy Mucus.**		
Mentals and Generals (see texts)	Also in long standing catarrhs with loss of smell in a mild, timid person. **A weepy** patient **demanding attention, sympathy & company. Changeability** of symptoms & states.	Catarrhs may alternate with joint pains.	May be weepy & depressed but want to be alone; hates fuss. May love or hate salt.	Weak & frail people, normally chilly.

Nose & sinuses

Remedy	Hepar sulph.	Mercurius	Euphrasia	Nux vomica
Cause & onset	Cold dry winds.	Cold & damp.		**Cold dry** winds or weather.
Site				
Sensations	Coryza with sneezing every time he goes in a cold wind; hypersensitive to **touch, pain & draughts of cold air**. Nose stuffs up in cold air, > heat.	**Rawness; burning;** sensation of pressure through bones of the face (sinusitis); swelling inside nose; sneezing a lot; **creeping chilliness**.	A burning, bruising, pressure pain in eyes like from dust with discharge from the eyes; swollen nasal mucous membranes; sneezing.	Nose stuffed & dry initially; nose **stuffed at night & in open air; chilly**, he hugs the fire; throat rough, raw, sore; sneezing.
Modalities	< Cold or uncovering, cold air. > Heat, moist wet weather.	< **Night, heat or cold, draughts,** sweating.	< Night (coryza), day (cough), open air & wind, lying down. > Night & lying down (cough).	< Morning, least **draught** or air movement, dry weather, warm room (coryza) before the fever comes on when he must have heat.
Discharges	**Smells sour or like decomposed cheese;** initially watery, later thick, yellow, offensive; profuse discharges.	**Thick, green or yellow, acrid, stinking.** Bloody; offensive. Thin & acrid at first, later thick & more bland.	**Bland nasal catarrh & acrid tears** indicates this remedy (opposite to *All c.*); cheeks sore from it. Severe fluent coryza tends to go down to larynx with a loud cough.	Fluent in warm room & by day; nose stuffed up at night & in open air.
Concomitants	Gets hoarse & coughs from every dry cold wind; may sweat all night without relief.	Fluent, **acrid** coryza, nose red & swollen, shining; much sneezing; mouth ulcers; hoarse voice; dry rough tickling cough. **Taste** metallic, sweet, salty, putrid. Increased **salivation; swollen flabby** tongue & gums; profuse, offensive **sweats**.	Catarrhs with **headaches**-bursting, bruised & lights dazzle; coryza extends to larynx with a hard cough; no cough at night like *Bryonia*.	Shivering from slightest motion or uncovering; chills alternate with heat; sweats easily; colds may go to the chest; dull head; may have a digestive upset too < eating.
Peculiars		Metallic taste.		
Mentals and Generals (see texts)	**Oversensitive to cold, touch & pain; chilly**, irritable person; always taking cold.	**Creeping chilliness;** trembling; must get up & walk the floor.	A chilly person; in fevers the **chills** predominate.	**Irritable; chilliness** of whole body not > warmth, cannot stir from the fire; oversensitive, touchy; sensitive to the least draught.

Nose & sinuses

Remedy	Gelsemium	Arsenicum	Rhus tox.	Ipecacuanha
Cause & onset	Warm moist mild weather; several days after exposure. **Slowly.**		Cold & damp weather; suppressed sweat. Onset at night.	Rapid onset.
Site				
Sensations	Sore nostrils as if hot water passing down them.	Sore nose & **burning; nose stuffed up all the time; sneezing** without relief of irritation; sneezes from every change of weather.	Nose stopped up with every cold; sore nostrils; thirst for cold drinks especially at night but may cause chilliness & cough; bones **ache, bruised & sore**; sneezing; tickling behind upper sternum.	Simple colds, settle in nose; **sneezing** excessively, causes blood in mucus. Colds begin in nose & spread rapidly to chest; stopped nose at night; violent chill, shakes all over & teeth chatter; no thirst.
Modalities		< Cold > Heat except the head > cool.	< Evening & night, **cold, damp**, uncovering, **rest & first movement** (pains). > **Heat**, continued movement (pains), perspiration.	< Damp. > Open air, rest.
Discharges	Acrid discharge, sore nostrils as if red hot water passing down them; watery discharge.	**Thin, watery, acrid coryza; sore upper lip.** He is happier when the discharge is thicker.	Violent coryza; thick yellow or green very offensive mucus.	Mucous discharge.
Concomitants	Teasing tickling cough > near fire; headache, congested head; occipital pain; face flushed & dusky, mottled; cold extremites, hot head.		Red swollen throat; sore throat with swollen glands & stiff neck. Hoarseness, rawness, roughness. Cough; colds settle throughout the limbs & body; dizzy.	Overwhelming **nausea with a clean tongue.** Violent chills; face flushed. colds descend causing hoarseness, rawness & on to the chest.
Peculiars		Feeling of ice cold in blood vessels in chills & boiling in fever. Burning > heat.	**Triangular red tip to tongue.**	Nosebleeds with every cold.
Mentals and Generals (see texts)	**Weight & tiredness; chills up & down the spine;** trembling weakness.	Always taking colds; **chilly,** suffers from a draught & hugs the fire; **burning pains** > **heat**; restless; anxious; thirst for ice cold in sips; **miserable**, weak & everything is extreme, out of proportion.	Fear & restless at night. Aches & pains < first motion, > continued motion but he tires.	Prostration comes in spells, not continous.

Nose & sinuses

(See also *Aconite, Calcarea, Eupator. perf., Ferrum phos., Kali carb., Lach., Lyc.* and *Spongia* for further possibilities)

Remedy	Sulphur	Allium cepa	Bryonia	Dulcamara
Cause & onset	**Later stages or if a cold lingers.** May easily take cold.	Cold, damp, penetrating winds.	Taking cold; cold, dry winds; suppressing a sweat. In morning.	Sudden change of weather, **hot to cold**; taking cold. Spring & Autumn colds.
Site		Left side then right.		
Sensations	**Burning anywhere**; congested, wants fresh air; constant sneezing; stoppage of the nose.	**Rawness; sneezing comes early** & with increasing frequency. Watery nasal discharge **burns the upper lip** like fire until **red & raw**; congested nose with sense of **fullness**, throbbing & burning; blocked stuffed up nose, goes from left to right.	**Stitching pains; dry** mouth; **Thirsty for large quantities of cold water** at long intervals. Complaints often start with sneezing, coryza, headache & red eyes.	Nose stuffs up in every spell of cold, damp weather.
Modalities	< 12 am & 12 pm, heat.	< Evening, warmth, indoors (coryza). > Outdoors (coryza).	< 9 pm, **motion, heat.** > Pressure, still.	< Evening & night, **cold & damp weather**, cold. > Heat, motion.
Discharges	**Acrid & burning**	**Bland watery eye discharge with acrid nasal discharge** indicates this remedy; **often both are profuse**.	Discharge is not so profuse; thick discharge. Eyes water red & sore.	Thick yellow mucus; bloody crusts.
Concomitants	Feels weak & hungry at 11 am; tired & slow convalescence.	Coryza may go to ears, larynx & throat; usually a catarrhal, congestive hadache; nosebleeds.	Miserable **headache**, headache accompanies most complaints; eyes red sore & watery; goes down onto chest; dry & painful cough.	Sore eyes from taking cold; ulcers of mucous membranes; back & neck pain & stiffness from cold & damp.
Peculiars				
Mentals and Generals (see texts)	Cannot take a bath, become overheated or get into a cold place without geting a cold.		< **Motion, want to be still & left alone**. Many complaints start with sneezing, coryza, red eyes & headache; may go to the throat, larynx & chest.	Recurrent colds; **marked** < **cold & damp.**

§8 Throat complaints

Remedy	Aconite	Belladonna	Arsenicum	Lycopodium
Cause & onset	Cold of draughts; cold dry wind. **Sudden onset.**	Cold. **Sudden onset.**	Always taking colds.	Slow onset.
Site		Right side especially.		**Right** to left or right side. May extend to ears.
Sensations	**Severe** pain; burning, tearing, rough scraping; painful swallowing; smarting; tingling; most painful. **Great thirst & dryness**; everything tastes bitter; spasms in the throat, as if choking; cannot swallow.	**Severe, burning** like coals of fire; **dry** spasmodic constriction, clutching, may be brought on by swallowing which is very painful; sensation of a lump; raw & sore; throbbing. **Great dryness & often great thirst**; desires lemonade, may be thirstless.	**Burning** pains; rough, scraping; hard cough. **Dry**, rasping throat with **thirst for frequent sips** of ice cold water.	Raw & sore; extremely painful; sensation of a lump; stitches on swallowing; dryness.
Modalities	< Warmth, warm room, covering up.	< 3 pm, night, **cold drinks**, open air, motion, **jar**, touch.	< Cold, change of weather, draughts, cold drinks. > **Heat (burning pains > heat)**, warm drinks.	< 4–8 pm, cold air, cold drinks. > **Warm drinks** usually.
Concomitants	**Violent high fever**; high grade inflammation, **very red**; red congested face.	**High fever**, hot head cold limbs; delirium with jerking & starting; dilated pupils; **redness or face** may later grow dusky; **red & swollen throat**, tonsils especially on right side; red strawberry tongue; **throbbing** carotids & headache; enlarged sore glands; aphthous ulcers, fine pin-head ulcers which may bleed; constant scraping & hawking of mucus; white coryza with much sneezing.	**Chilliness**, even during the fever, which is not usually high; throat may look red & shrivelled; frequently **ulcerated**, may bleed easily. Tickling hard cough; usually has coryza with sneezing.	Swollen tongue; food & drink may tend to regurgitate into the nose on swallowing; blocked nose; congested head which he wants uncovered & cool.
Peculiars	Bitter taste.		**Burning > heat.**	
Mentals and Generals (see texts)	**Anxiety**, fear, restlessness; everything is intense & violent, not lingering. May normally be a vigorous healthy plethoric person.	Rapid progress & onset. Starts & jumps in delirious high fever. **Not** used in lingering states.	**Chilly, anxious, restless, prostrate**; sinking & disproportionately weak. Tends to go down onto the chest with constriction & a dry hacking cough.	Usually not very sick; desire fresh air.

Throat complaints

Remedy	Arnica	Hepar sulph.	Nitric acid	Phytolacca
Cause & onset	Overexertion.	Dry cold wind.	Takes cold easily.	
Site		Extends to ears.		Extends to ears. Root of tongue.
Sensations	Raw & sore; dry & thirsty; thirst only during the chill.	Of a **splinter**, of something stuck in the throat. A lump, a **swelling** in the throat. **Very chilly; severe throbbing pains**; painful swallowing; throat very sensitive to touch.	Of a **splinter** of something stuck in the throat; stinging & burning pains with a sore mouth; raw & sore. **Very chilly**; usually thirstless even in the fever; swallowing causes violent pains which can go to the ears; dysphagia & choking; draws head down when he swallows.	**Splinter** pains; sore, dry, rough, burning, smarting; incessant desire to swallow which is painful & may extend to the ears. Pain in the **root of the tongue on protrusion. Chilly** & desires to be covered. Sensation of a lump on swallowing saliva; throat full as if choked.
Modalities	< Touch, motion, jar.	< **Cold**. uncovering, slightest draught. **Touch**, pressure. > Warm drinks, heat.	< **Cold**, touch.	< Night, **warm drinks**, heat of bed, cold days, swallowing.
Concomitants	Head hot, body cold; **great bodily soreness** which makes him restless & the bed feel hard.	**Marked swelling of throat & tonsils**; suppuration of tonsils, quinsy even; dusky purple colour; copious catarrh with a foul cheesy odour; perspiration at night without relief.	**Swelling** of uvula & tonsils, oedematous; yellow exudate in patches on tonsils; red or purple inflammation; foul odour; ragged, jagged **ulcers**; white or dark putrid bleeding; saliva is acrid; viscid mucus in throat. Urine very strong, smells like a horse's.	Swelling of tonsils; great **swelling of throat; dark red**, even bluish or purplish; low grade inflammation; coated tongue; thick tenacious mucus; ulceration; **glands swollen & hard**, especially submaxillary & parotids.
Peculiars		Uncovering even a hand increases the pain & cough.		Acute pain at base of tongue on protrusion.
Mentals and Generals (see texts)	Wants to be left alone, not talked to; nightmares; says he is all right. See *Fevers*.	Irritable & easily angered; touchy; hypersensitive senses. Chronically enlarged tonsils. Not usually used early in an illness.	Recurrent coryza. Usually is chilly & may love salt & fat foods.	**Much aching in the body**, may cause restlessness which < the pains. **Breast complaints**. Spasms, cramps & drawing pains.

Throat complaints

Remedy	Sulphur	Pulsatilla	Phosphorus	Silica
Cause & onset	Change of weather or air. Lingering states.	Getting wet, especially feet.	Overheating; changes of weather.	Cold, getting wet. Very slow onset, after a series of colds.
Site				
Sensations	**Burning pains**; raw, stitching, pressing, cutting, splinter, rough, scraping. Painful difficult swallowing; sensation of **swelling**, of a lump, a splinter or a hair; sensitive throat; **dry mucous membranes, thirsty**.	Rough scraping; constriction & tickling caused cough. Sensation of a lump; stinging pains < swallowing saliva. **Thirstless** despite a **dry mouth**; bad taste especially in the morning. Pains with chilliness.	Intense **burning**, extends to oesophagus even; rough, scraping, raw, sore pains; constriction. **Thirst for cold; great dryness**; violent hunger. Sensation of cotton or velvet in throat; larynx very sensitive to touch or cold; unable to swallow.	Splinter pains; stinging pain on swallowing.
Modalities	< 12 am & pm, night, heat.	< **Warmth**, stuffy rooms, fats. > **Open cool air**, gentle motion.	< Evening, **warm to cold air**, talking, coughing, eating.	
Concomitants	Purple aspect or dusky tonsils; swollen tonsils; suppuration with purplish tonsils. **Catarrhal states**; ulceration; redness round orifices of the body.	**Yellow/green, bland discharges** from anywhere; profuse; catarrh of throat. Throat bluish red; veins distended; coated tongue; flushes to the face.	Laryngitis with hoarseness < evening; larynx so painful he cannot talk & suppresses coughing; much swelling of tonsils & uvula; copious salivation, tastes sweet, salty or foul; sore excoriated bleeding mouth even.	Sweat of head & neck; catarrhal throat with hoarseness, chronic catarrh; flushes of heat, fever with cold extremities; glands enlarged & sore, swollen parotids; suppuration & quinsy.
Peculiars				
Mentals and Generals (see texts)	**Lingering sore throats; lethargy** & may hate standing. Offensive breath, sweat & discharges.	Changeable symptoms. **Mild, gentle, tearful, clingy** etc. Wants fuss & help.		Colds settle in the throat; overheats easily & suffocates in a warm room in an acute illness, normally chilly & < draughts; may be needed after *Pulsatilla*.

Throat complaints

Remedy	Carbo veg.	Rhus tox.	Bryonia	Natrum mur.
Cause & onset	Overheating.	**Cold & damp,** suppressed sweat. Overuse of the voice.	Cold especially if overheated. Slow onset.	Takes cold easily while sweating. 10–11 am.
Site				
Sensations	Scraping, rawness, smarting; cannot swallow food because so sore; feels swollen; dryness; bad tasting mucus. Becomes hoarse & a cough develops.	**Sore pain;** sensation of swelling; dry mucous membranes, **violent thirst** for cold drinks which may chill; painful first swallowing.	Stitching & nondescript pains. **Parched dry & great thirst** for large volumes at long intervals; cold drinks may bring on a cough.	**Splinter pains** on swallowing; **stitching, shooting** pains; sensation of a lump; **thirst for cold; extreme dryness** of mucus membranes, when not covered by catarrhal mucus; food sticks all the way & must be washed down.
Modalities		< Morning. **Cold,** first motion. > **Heat, warm drinks,** continued motion.	< 9 pm, **motion,** heat. > Cold.	< 10–11 am, change of weather. > Sweat.
Concomitants	**Copious watery nasal discharge. Bleeding.** Later get yellow/green discharge; fever evening & night; **cold sweat,** sweats in a warm room, chilled by the cold; cold skin; great pallor & **coldness,** breath may even be cold. Purple aphthous ulcers, ooze black blood & run together.	Swollen glands & neck; stiff neck. Triangular red tip to the tongue; dry or coated.	**Headache** precedes or accompanies nearly all complaints; bursting congestive headache < slightest motion, light, noise, cough. Thickly coated white tongue; aphthous ulcers.	Dryness without ulceration or a catarrhal discharge like egg white; red, swollen, oedematous; mouth feels dry even if wet; dry cracked lips; crack in centre of lips; cold sores about lips.
Peculiars	**Cold yet desires to be fanned.**		.	Thirst for cold drinks even during the chill.
Mentals and Generals (see texts)	Often starts with a coryza from being overheated. Face flushes after wine.	**Restless;** less tired & more achy than *Arsenicum.* Anxious, irritable & weepy.	Irritable, does not want to talk; **wants to be left alone in peace;** may be stuporose in a fever.	Takes cold easily while sweating. Often a very sensitive, easily offended patient.

Throat complaints

Remedy	Nux vomica	Chamomilla	Mercurius	Lachesis
Cause & onset	Cold dry winds. Takes cold very easily.	Taking cold. Evenings often.	Taking cold.	Taking cold; going from cold to warm.
Side	Stitches into the ear.			**Left or left to right.** Pain in root of tongue, goes to ears.
Sensations	Rough scraping pain, raw & sore; tightness & tension, constricted sensation; dry, tickly cough. **Chilly, sensitive to the least draught**; great heat but cannot uncover without feeling chilly.	**Severe pain.** Sore, spasms, constrictions & pain as if from a plug; usually thirsty for cold drinks.	**Severe stinging**; raw & sore, smarting. Difficult swallowing from pain & paralytic weakness; tongue feels swollen. **Great dryness** though may appear wet; thirst; sweet, salty, metallic, foul taste. Ulcers sting & burn. Sore throat with every cold.	**Severe pains. Throat very sensitive to touch,** even clothing on the neck may cause choking sensation; raw burning & splinter pains; sensation of a lump, a constriction; very painful swallowing yet has desire to swallow; difficulty swallowing; chokes & gags on warm things; **extreme dryness without thirst.**
Modalities	< Cold, draughts, uncovering; heat before the fever. > Heat (with fever).	< 9 am, 9–12 pm, night, heat. > Being carried.	< Night, **heat or cold**, draught, sweating.	< **On waking**, am, **heat, warm drinks,** empty swallowing, drinking, light touch. > Pressure, swallowing solids, sometimes by cold drinks.
Concomitants	Thin watery coryza by day; sneezing from itching in the nose; very red face with fever; digestive upset, sour stomach or constipation.	**Marked swelling**; uniform redness; swollen parotid & submaxillary glands; poor appetite.	**Salivation** & drools, yet feels dry & thirsty; **offensive** mouth; **swollen** throat, **glands** & tongue flabby taking the imprint of the teeth; tongue thick, yellow & moist; still neck; **suppuration, quinsy** or throat looks red & pale as if will suppurate; white or yellow exudate; ulcers with a lardaceous base; **sweating** profuse does not relieve; thick yellow/green offensive nasal discharge.	Throat **swollen** or feels it; bluish red, mottled purple. Purple congested puffy face; stringy, sticky saliva. Red grey deep aphthous ulcers, especially on margins of mucus membranes. Swollen glands & muscles of neck inflamed & tender. Paralysis of pharynx causing gagging & choking. Suppuration from right to left.
Peculiars				May swallow solids easier than liquids, > even.
Mentals and Generals (see texts)	Oversensitive, irritable, chilly.	**Great irritability**; cannot control temper; sensitive to pain; capricious, nothing pleases etc. The emotional state will usually indicate this remedy.	Weakness. Sensitive to heat & cold; offensiveness of odours; trembling. **Do not give early in the illness or repeat too often.**	**Surgings** of blood. Chokings when going to sleep or on waking; chronic sore throats; soreness in back of head & neck.

Throat complaints

(See also *Calcarea, Dulcamara, Kali bich.* and *Spongia* for further possibilities)

Argentum nit.	Apis	Lac. caninum	Gelsemium	Merc. cyan.
	Emotion, jealousy, anger. Quite rapid onset.		Several days after exposure to cold moist mild winters. **Slow onset.**	
	Right or right to left.	**Changes sides**. Goes to left ear.		
Splinter pains; raw, sore, rough & scraping; strangulated feeling. Desires cold drinks.	**Stinging, burning** pains; splinter pains; raw & sore; constriction of throat; usually **thirstless**.	Splinter pain, sore; oversensitive, hyper-aesthesia; throat closing & sensation as if will choke; very sensitive to external touch, swallowing nearly impossible. Throat dry, husky.	Sore, comes on gradually; hot skin, high fever; chills up & down the back, as if rubbed with ice, causes shuddering.	Raw & sore.
< Warmth, cold drinks.	< **Heat, hot drinks**, radiant heat.	< Empty swallowing.		
> Fresh air.	> **Cold, cold drinks.**	> Cold or warm drinks.	> Lying with the head high, propped up.	
Much thick mucous catarrh in the throat with loss of voice; dark red throat, swollen; ulcerated.	**Marked swelling, oedema** of uvula; throat, tonsils, tongue; oedema looks as if full of water; **red**. Fever with chills yet still < heat. Slowly progressive exudate on tonsils; ulcers. Dry hot skin alternates with perspiration; thirstless; rashes, dry and rough; scanty urine.	Coryza with sneezing. Glazed shiny red appearance; ulcers appear dry & glistening; felt-like exudate, silvery grey shiny deposit; paralysis of the throat with nasal regurgi-tation of food & drink.	Red tonsils; high fever with cold extremities; muscular weakness generally, tired & heavy; nasal regurgitation from weakness of muscles.	Throat looks raw in spots, as if denuded; broken down appearance of mucus membranes, bordering on suppuration. Follicular tonsillitis.
		Cannot bear the touch of her own skin.		
Desires cold room & cold air. Nervous & impulsive, may have a sweet tooth.	**Face flushed; suffocation from heat**. Scarlet fever.	Full of imagining, harrassing, tormenting thoughts; hysterical even; very sensitive; may see spiders, snakes, vermin. Cannot bear to be alone; may think she has a terrible disease.	**Great weight & tiredness of body & limbs.**	See *Mercurius* for the rest of the symptoms.

Throats: When to seek advice

Urgently, Right now!

- If the throat is so severely swollen as to cause difficulty breathing.
- If the pain is very severe with inability to swallow and much drooling.
- If there is bleeding from the mouth with measles.

Within 24 hours

- If unusual and very marked swelling occurs around the tonsils on one or both sides.
- Severe sore throats persisting more than a day or two in a young child without signs of improvement.
- If there has been a history of rheumatic fever in the past.

Refer to other chapters as necessary.

§9 Abdominal complaints

Remedy	Aconite	Belladonna	Colocynthis	Chamomilla
Cause & onset	Taking cold or in very hot weather. **Sudden onset.**	Chill.	Anger, indignation, taking offence, rich foods; drinking when overheated.	
Sensations	Shooting, burning, stinging pains; weight in stomach; flatulent colic.	Colic is like *Colocynth*. burning, griping, distension, violent colics. **Appear & disappear suddenly.**	**Colics**, violent **clutching, cramping, grasping pains**; tearing; paroxysms of increasing severity until he vomits; agonising; passes flatus which >.	**Colic** especially in infants, doubles up, kicks & screams; cutting, burning, griping pains; distension after eating.
Modalities (General)	< Touch.	< **Jar**, motion, pressure, lying on the affected side. > Bending forward.	< **At rest** – drives to despair but pains < motion, eating or drinking. > **Doubling up, hard pressure, heat**, lying on stomach, belching or flatus.	< Eructations. > Heat maybe.
Diarrhoea	Great tenesmus; dysentery of blood & a little slime; nausea & perspiration before diarrhoea; green stools.	Frequent urging to stool with little or no result.	With the pains; frequent & excessive urging to stool; severe diarrhoea; **flatulence**; mucous stools in dysentery.	**Grass green or like chopped eggs**, with grass green mucus; feels hot as it passes; smells of rotten eggs; diarrhoea with teething.
Modalities (Diarrhoea)			< Slight eating. > Heat.	
Nausea & vomiting	Awful, retching too; vomiting of bright red blood; **violent & sudden** nausea & vomiting; desire pungent or bitter things yet everything tastes bitter.		Vomits with the pain, often no preceding nausea, may just retch.	Much vomiting; eructations smell of rotten eggs; violent retching with cold sweat; salivation; putrid breath.
Modalities (Nausea & vomiting)				
Concomitants	Febrile state.	Hot head & cold extremities; face red.	**Coated tongue**	
Mentals and Generals (see texts)	Anguish, restless anxiety; red face; thirst etc.	Marked fever, thirst & redness etc. Dilated pupils; < draught.	**Irritable & angry**; they want instant pain relief. **Extreme restlessness & weak** with the pain; faint; dizzy; wants to be alone.	Very irritable, restless, oversensitive, hard to please etc. Moans & howls; they do **not** bear pain calmly & patiently!

Abdominal complaints

Remedy	Mag. phos.	Ipecacuanha	Nux vomica	Phosphorus
Cause & onset	Cold, cold damp weather. Sudden pains.	Overeating; rich foods. Suppressed emotion; pregnancy. **Rapid onset.**	**Overeating; excess stimulants;** overwork.	Stormy weather.
Sensations	**Colic**, in infants; spasms in stomach with a **clean tongue; cramps**; radiating pains; distension & much flatulence; nipping, griping, pinching; intense cramps & cutting; restless.	**Tenesmus**; griping pains especially at the umbilicus; colic with nausea & green stools; sharp pains in gastritis; pains between the scapulae; distended stomach.	Colicky pains shoot from or to the rectum, upwards from rectum; rending, tearing, cutting, pain with tenesmus; bends double. Putrid bitter taste in mouth but food & drink are O.K.; distension & tenderness; pressure pain, sensation of a weight in stomach; flatulence.	**Burning pains**; pressing, tearing; distension; **thirst for cold**; may have a hungry empty feeling, must eat or will faint.
Modalities (General)	< Night, stretched out, cold, touch, motion. > **Heat & warm applications, doubling up, hard pressure**, rubbing. Not > belching.	< Overeating.	< Morning (with foul mouth like *Puls.*). **Eating, cold,** motion, slightest pressure. > Heat, rest, sitting or lying.	< Evening, **warm things**, touch. > **Cold things.**
Diarrhoea		Green, slimy, watery, bloody; profuse or slight; fermented, foamy. Burning & tenesmus.	Tenesmus; much **straining but scanty stool** which >; ineffectual urge to stool; **constipation** usually.	Gurgling down the gut leads to diarrhoea; profuse; bloody; foetid, gushing stools; lumps of white mucus. Cramps & burning in anus; **tenesmus**; sensation as if anus is wide open.
Modalities (Diarrhoea)			> Passing a stool.	
Nausea & vomiting		**Constant nausea marks this remedy.** Vomits everything taken. Vomiting of bile with a **clean tongue** or only slight coating; empty eructations & salivation; nausea in morning. Nausea which nothing relieves.	**Much retching & straining & effort** before is able to vomit; eating causes uneasiness; bitter & sour eructations; constant nausea, no appetite.	Vomiting of warm drinks, > cold drinks but may be vomited once they become warm in stomach. Eructations of food or gas.
Modalities (Nausea & vomiting)		< Overeating. > Open air, rest.	< Morning, after eating. > Evening.	< Warm things are vomited immediately. > **Cold things** which may be vomited when they warm in stomach.
Concomitants	**Clean tongue**. Right sided.	**Clean tongue.**	Bursting crushing vertex headache with stomach upset.	Hunger at 11 am.
Mentals and Generals (see texts)	Twitching of muscles; cramps, more sensitive to a cold draught; thin, tense anxious & chilly (unlike *Colocynth.*).	Prostration in spells; pallor or red & congested etc. Sulky, despises everything.	Chilly & oversensitive; angry & easily offended; sensitive to noise, odour, light etc. Irritable.	Bleeding & bruising. > for a short sleep.

Abdominal complaints

Remedy	Lycopodium	Silica	Sulphur	Arsenicum
Cause & onset	Seafood.	Diarrhoea from overheating.		
Sensations	Sensation of **fullness, belching & flatulence; distended with flatus** often after eating just a little; gnawing, burning pains; pressure & heaviness, must loosen clothing; noisy rumblings.	Soreness from pressure; colic & flatulence.	**Burning**, soreness; sensation of a **weight** in stomach, after eating; distension; flatulence & colic with no wind; hunger, may drink little but eat much; congestion.	Burning > heat. Stitching pains; stomach very sensitive to touch; violent pains with great anguish; distension; **thirst for sips of cold.**
Modalities (General)	< **4–8 pm, after eating, cold things**, pressure. > **Warm drinks.**	< **Pressure of clothes,** after eating. > **Heat.**	< 12 am & 12 pm, heat, after eating.	< Touch, cold drinks. > Heat except head.
Diarrhoea	All kinds of diarrhoea, the other symptoms will distinguish this remedy.	Sour curds in stool; changeable like *Pulsatilla*; during hot weather or dentition.	Early morning diarrhoea, drives him from his bed. Sore anus with diarrhoea – burns & raw; offensive; tenesmus.	Stools burn; frequent urging with tenesmus; involuntary stool; stools acrid, putrid odours; dysentery with bloody diarrhoea.
Modalities (Diarrhoea)	< 4–8 pm.	< Milk.	< 5 am.	< After midnight.
Nausea & vomiting	Vomits bile or coffee grounds; sour, burning eructations; noisy rumblings; nervous dyspepsia, heartburn & waterbrash.	Sour vomiting. Weak stomach in old dyspeptics.	All gone hungry feeling especially at 11 am; sensitive to touch; acid, bilious acrid vomiting; sour reflux.	Vomiting of everything taken; a little warm water may relieve then is vomited; painful vomiting; gastritis; diarrhoea & vomiting simultaneously.
Modalities (Nausea & vomiting)	< 4–8 pm.	< Milk.	< 12 am & 12 pm, after eating.	< Eating or drinking, cold drinks.
Concomitants	Loses appetite soon after starting to eat or vice versa and gains it.	Averse to milk.		Dry mouth & thirst for sips.
Mentals and Generals (see texts)	**Flatulence & belching, fullness** with little appetite etc.		Poor digestion, faint & weak if does not eat; < heat; intolerant of clothing & its weight; likes sweets, fat, alcohol, beer normally.	Chilly, pale, restless, prostrate out of proportion; anxiety & fears etc. < Cold & night.

Abdominal complaints

Remedy	Veratrum a.	Podophyllum	China	Bryonia
Cause & onset		Summer diarrhoea of children.	Diarrhoea at night.	Taking cold; overheating, especially if takes cold drinks; dietary excesses.
Sensations	Twisting, griping, **forced to bend double** which does not help; burning in pit of stomach with great sinking feeling.	**Cramping pains which double him up** & rumblings preceding stool which usually >; rectum sore & may prolapse; empty, all gone, weak sensation; dragging down.	**Bloated, distension to bursting not relieved by belching.** Constant loud eructations; sore bowels, cannot move.	Stitching, sore, tender, burning; disordered stomach; distended abdomen, sensation as if it would burst; very sensitive to touch & pressure; weight in stomach after eating; thirst.
Modalities (General)		< Pressure (very sore).	< Motion, touch, cold.	< **motion**, eating, touch, pressure (lies with legs drawn up).
	> Walking.	> Lying on abdomen, passing stool.	> Warmth, pressure.	> Applied heat.
Diarrhoea	**Diarrhoea & vomiting simultaneously**; purging until **exhausted; copious stool**; watery, green, colourless, great mass of stool.	**Very explosive diarrhoea** with flatus; so profuse she may faint; offensive, copious, frequent, gushing, gurgling, wattery diarrhoea; painless; bright yellow.	Copious diarrhoea; painless.	Yellow mushy stool or dry & hard constipation; diarrhoea preceded by cutting pains in abdomen; daytime.
Modalities (Diarrhoea)		< 4 am, after bathing, acid or tinned fruit, milk.	< Night, after eating.	< Morning on beginning to move. **Motion.**
Nausea & vomiting	**Diarrhoea & vomiting simultaneously**; forcible & excessive vomiting.	Gagging; eructations smelling of bad eggs.	Hiccough, nausea & vomiting; bitter, sour eructations; bitter, salty, exaggerated taste.	Bitter nauseating taste; bilious vomiting; dry mouth with **thirst**; nausea on waking.
Modalities (Nausea & vomiting)			< Night, fruit, wine, fish, milk.	< **Motion**, after eating, sitting up. > Lying still & flat.
Concomitants	Cold sweat on forehead	Diarrhoea with liver pains.		Thickly coated white tongue.
Mentals and Generals (see texts)	**Great cold sweat; coldness; blueness.** Very rapid onset of weakness; **prostration**; cramps.	Thirst for cold water; may be drowsy & desire to stretch all the time; prostration.		Wants to be left alone, in peace; irritable; does not want to talk or think.

Abdominal complaints

Remedy	Natrum sulph.	Pulsatilla	Gelsemium	Ant. tart.
Cause & onset	Wet weather.	Rich foods.	Anticipation, emotional upsets.	**Sour** food fruit or wine. Rapid prostration.
Sensations	**Fullness** & sense of **distension; flatus** with **rumbling & gurgling; wind pains.**	Bloating; colicky pains; rumbling; very tender; sensation of weight in stomach, dragging down, drawing pain; cutting, **flitting, changeable pains;** bad taste, dry mouth yet thirstless.		Distended with flatulence; often just felt as an anxiety in the stomach; colicky, cutting pains too. Usually thirstless but may desire cold or sour things which are vomited.
Modalities (General)	> Flatus & belching.	< **Morning, heat, rich fatty foods.** > **Fresh air, cold,** gentle motion.		
Diarrhoea	Diarrhoea with mucus on rising; feeling as if diarrhoea would come on but passes only flatus; gushing thin diarrhoea, often painless.	**Loose, watery, green, ever changeing stool; no two ever alike;** alternates with constipation; flatulence; mucus stools, soft; little blood.	Sudden diarrhoea from nervous anticipation, emotion; involuntary stool or urine from paralysis during a fever.	
Modalities (Diarrhoea)	< Morning, evening.	< **Evening & night, keeping still.** > **Gentle motion.**		
Nausea & vomiting	Bitter eructations; slimy, bitter taste; bitter vomiting.	Eructations of bitter food, bile < in evening; bad taste < morning; diminished sense of taste.		**Constant nausea & deadly loathing of food;** averse to milk – is vomited; vomits cold or sour things; violent retching, straining, gagging to vomit; vomits lots of mucus; tenacious, white, ropy, stringy slime; later bile & with all the straining, blood.
Modalities (Nausea and vomiting)		< Morning, fatty rich foods.		Vomiting > nausea unlike *Ipecac.*
Concomitants		**Thirstlessness with dryness;** coated tongue.	Dim, double or misty vision before headache.	
Mentals and Generals (see texts)	Generally < heat & humid weather.	**Clingy, weepy, changeable etc.**	Ptosis, thirstless, weak.	Irritable, cold, pale & prostrate; feeble & broken down; aversion to being touched or even looked at, wants to be let alone.

Abdominal complaints

(See also *Apis, Calcarea, Eupator. perf., Kali bich., Merc.* and *Nat. mur.* for further possibilities

Dulcamara	Sepia	Ant. crud.	Carbo. veg.	Dioscorea
Diarrhoea from taking **cold** when hot, going from hot to cold, from cold **damp**.	Pregnancy.	Sour wine; eating what disagrees; summer diarrhoea.		
Colic as if diarrhoea would come on; tearing cutting pains before stool.	Faint sinking empty all gone feeling in pit of stomach not > by eating; bearing down pains in pelvis; stitches & burning; rumbling flatulent distension.	Loathing for food & drink; may desire acids & pickles which >; sensation of a lump in stomach, feels overloaded, distended; burning pains; thirstless.	Constricting & cramping pains from distension with gas; a fullness; belching sour disordered stomach; burning; flatulent; offensive sweat; raw around anus.	Severe cutting, frequent colic pains; griping, rumbling & passes a lot of wind; pains radiate to distant parts, come & go, reappear in a different place; pains can shoot; colic not usually > stool; mouth dry & bitter.
	Pain < vomiting.		< Lying down, pressure. > **Belching.**	< **Doubling up,** lying. > **Stretching** out or standing straight, motion, walking in open air.
Infantile diarrhoea; no digestion; changeable stools like *Puls.*; often yellow & watery.	Diarrhoea from milk; chronic diarrhoea with jelly like lumpy stools; much mucus; very offensive.	Lumpy & liquid diarrhoea; passes little & often, later gets tenesmus.	Diarrhoea & flatulence; putrid; very offensive; bloody watery stools; mucus.	In early morning, drives him from bed; yellowish; burning.
< **Cold damp weather.**				< Morning.
	Morning nausea either < or > eating; nausea from smell of food or cooking; sour & bitter eructations of food; vomiting of mucus & bile; empty all gone feeling.	Catarrh, nausea & vomiting; constant nausea; retching after vomiting which does not >.	Constant eructations & regurgitation; all food taken seems to turn to wind.	Sour eructations; sinking at the pit of the stomach.
			> **Belching.**	
		Thick milky white coating on tongue.	Cold sweat; face flushes after a little wine.	
Catarrhs < cold damp etc.	Aversion to food, meat fat & bread. Indifferent, hates fuss & sympathy; flashes of heat with sweat & faintness.	Sentimental, peevish; dislikes even to be looked at.	**Coldness,** chilly; air hunger, wants to be fanned vigorously; sluggish lazy turgid, full swollen puffed; relaxed; pallor.	Irritable with the pains; depressed & averse to company.

Abdomen: When to seek advice

Urgently, Right now!

- If there are significant signs of dehydration (loss of body fluids), usually from diarrhoea or vomiting, especially in an infant, as shown by:
    1. Eyes appear sunken.
    2. In babies the fontanelle (soft spot on the top of the head) is sunken.
    3. Dryness of the mouth or eyes.
    4. Loss of skin tone or turgor – gently pinch up the skin which will normally snap straight back into place. If it does not then marked dehydration is present.
    5. Decreased quantity of urine being passed. It may be very strong.
- Constant repeated vomiting.
- If the vomit is bloodstained or looks like coffee grounds.
- If the stool is bloody, black or tar-like. Bleeding from the rectum with measles.
- If marked abdominal symptoms follow a head or abdominal injury, especially if vomiting follows a head injury (see First Aid Section).
- Severe pain anywhere in the abdomen.
- In children with vomiting, inconsolable screaming or lethargy.
- If there is evidence or suspicion of drugs or poisonous substances having been taken. If possible keep a sample of the substance and of the vomited material for later analysis.

Within 24 hours

- Unexpected swelling, pain or tenderness in the groin or insides of the tops of the thighs.
- For constipation with pain and or vomiting of a day or more duration.
- Abdominal symptoms in someone with diabetes may become urgent – advice should always be sought sooner for a person with diabetes.
- Likewise with abdominal symptoms in a pregnant lady – if in doubt, seek advice.
- Signs of jaundice – yellow eyes or skin, dark urine and there may be light coloured stools.
- Any urinary symptoms – pains, discharge, bleeding or deposit in the urine, frequent urging, especially if the urinary symptoms are accompanied by a backache or loin pains which may suggest that the kidneys are affected in some way.

Refer to other chapters as necessary.

§10 Coughs

The *Coughs* section has been arranged in the form of a table with the different characteristics of the cough in the lefthand column. The following symbols indicate their intensity or effect on the cough in each of the remedies:

± + and ++   **indicate mild, moderate and marked intensity**
> and >>   **indicate conditions under which the cough is improved and markedly improved**
< and <<   **indicate conditions which worsen and markedly worsen the cough**

An 'A' under the 'Thirst' section means that the thirst is usually absent.
The word 'from' indicates a cause of the cough.

When using this table you may find it easier to take a sheet of A4 paper, place it alongside the column of *Characteristics* and mark the symptoms of your patient on the edge of the sheet using the above symbols. You can then move the paper across the table and compare symptoms of the case to each remedy in turn and make a note of those that match the best. Choose your remedy from this list with reference to the *Materia Medica* and other tables as appropriate.

Coughs

(See also *Apis*, *Calcarea*, *Carbonica* and *Eupator. perf.* for further possibilities. Refer to other chapters as necessary.)

Characteristics	Aconite	Allium cepa	Ant. t	Arsenicum	Belladonna	Bryonia	Causticum	Drosera	Dulcamera	Euphrasia	Ferrum phos.	Gelsemium	Hepar sulph.	Ipecacuana
Sudden onset	+				+									+
Slow onset			+			+	+				±	+		
Loose		±	+	Later +		+			±	±	±		±	±
Dry	+	±		Early +	+	+	±	±	±	±	±	±	±	±
Morning				<<			<			<<			<	
Day					<	<				<<	<			
Night	<<			<<	<	>	<	<<	<	>>		<	<<	<<
Loose morning						+							+	
Dry morning			±			±	±						±	
Dry evening		±		+	+	±							+	
Dry night	±			+	+	±			+				+	+
Croupy	++	±		±	±				+			±	++	
Suffocating	±		+	±		±	±	+					+	+
Dry mouth	+		±	+	+	+	±		±		±	±		
Thirst	+ cold		A	+ cold	+	+			+	+		A		
Drinking				<	<		>	>	<<				<	
Drinks warm				>>		>>								
Drinks cold				<<			>					<		
Eating			<	<		<					<		<	<
Cold food		From <	From <										<	
Warmth	<	<<	<			<<		<<	<<	>			>	<
Cold				<<		From <	<		From <	From <	<	From	<<	
Cold damp weather		From <	From <						<<					<
Cold dry weather	From <<						<						<<	
Open air	<	< >		<<		>>		>	>	<<	<		<	>
Bathing														
Motion					<	<	<<			<<	<	Too weak		
Exertion														
Deep breathing				<<		<			<<		<		<	
Talking					<		<	<<		<	<		<	±
Lying down			<	<		<	<<	<<	<	>	<			<
Lying on left side								<						
Pressure on chest					<	>		>					<	
With **chest pains**	±				+	+		+		±	±			
With **throat pain**	±	+			+	±							±	
With **hoarseness**	++	+	±	±	+	±	++	++	+	±		±	+	±
With **cold sores**				±			±		±				±	±

Coughs

Characteristics	Kali bich.	Kali carb.	Lachesis	Lycopodium	Mercurius	Natrum mur.	Nux vomica	Phosphorus	Pulsatilla	Rhus tox.	Rumex	Spongia	Sulphur
Sudden onset													
Slow onset												±	
Loose		±	±	±	±			±	am +		±		±
Dry	±	+	+	±	±	+	+	+	pm +	±	±	+	+
Morning	<<	<<		<	<	<	<<	<<	<<		<<		<<
Day		<	<<	<				<<					<
Night		<<	<<	<<	<<	<		<	<<	<	<<	<	<<
Loose morning						±	±	±	+				+
Dry morning	±	+		±			±			+			±
Dry evening	±	+	±	+	±	±	+	+	+	+		+	+
Dry night		+	+	+	+	±	+	+	+	+		+	+
Croupy	+		+					+			±	++	
Suffocating		±	On waking				+	±	±			±	+
Dry mouth	+	±	+	+	+	+	+	+	±	+		+	+
Thirst			+		+	+ cold		+	A	+			+
Drinking		<>	<	<				<				>>	
Drinks warm				>>			>>			>>		>	
Drinks cold				<	<			<		<		<	
Eating	<<	<<		<			<<	<			<<	<	<
Cold food					<								
Warmth	>	>	<	<			>		<<			<<	<
Cold	<	<<	<				Dry <<	<<	>	From <<	<	From	<
Cold damp weather	<	<								From <			<
Cold dry weather							<<	<			<	<	
Open air		<	<	<				<<	>>	<	<<		<>
Bathing										<<			<
Motion	<	<		<	<		<	<	>		<		
Exertion		<		<	<	<	<	<<					<
Deep breathing	<		<	<	<			<	±		<	<	<
Talking			<		<			<			<<	<	<
Lying down	>	<	<	<	<			<		<<	<<		<
Lying on left side				<	<			<			<		<
Pressure on chest								>					
With **chest pain**	±	±				±	±	+	+	+	±	+	
With **throat pain**	±	±	±				±	+	±			±	
With **hoarseness**	+		±	±	±	±	±	+		+	+	+	
With **cold sores**							+			+		±	±

Coughs: When to seek advice

Urgently, Right now!

- If there is severe difficulty in breathing – shortness of breath, wheezing, laboured, rapid or shallow breathing.
- If the conscious level of the patient is affected – confusion, drowsiness.
- If there is marked chest pain.
- If something solid has been inhaled. There is likely to be much coughing, though not always and the coughing may cease. Help should be urgently sought.
- If the patient's lips, tongue or face take on a purply-bluish tint.

Within 24 hours

- If the cough persists without improvement for a week or more and there is much weakness, tiredness and lack of energy.
- If the breathing is laboured or rapid. If unexpected wheezing or chest pain occurs. Clearly the young the patient and the more severe the breathing difficulty the more urgent becomes the need for help.
- Significant cough for 4 or more days with no signs of improvement during measles.

Refer to other chapters as necessary.

§11 Cystitis

Whilst each episode of cystitis may be helped by remedies selected from these tables, the tendency for the condition to recur is unlikely to be affected. One of the constitutional forms of therapy would be of value in this situation. See *Conditions Requiring Constitutional Therapy* on page 137. Cystitis is relatively common in women. In men it is rare and should always be checked out with your health care practitioner because it may be an indication that there is something else wrong in the urinary system.

In general cystitis will be helped by drinking plenty of clear fluids. Pure water (such as bottled or filtered) is the best drink. Fresh vegetables, salads and sweet fruit are good. It is best to avoid or limit the intake of acid or acid producing foods and drinks such as those containing refined sugars, tea, coffee, alcohol, citrus fruits and juices etc, (although home-made lemon barley water is a useful traditional remedy.)

Acute cystitis is usually accompanied by excessive acidity in the body. *Natrum Phosphoricum* 6x three or four times a day given **as well as** the indicated remedy will often help the body to rectify this acid imbalance and hence helps the indicated remedy to work more effectively and quickly.

Cystitis

Remedy	Sarsaparilla	Natrum mur.	Ferrum phos.	Kali muriaticum
Cause & onset	From a chill. Cold wet weather.		Slow onset, often over several hours or a day or two. From cold or over-exertion.	
Sensations	Ineffectual desire to urinate or only dribbles away, sometimes better (>) for standing up. The urine may flood the bed in the night. Severe pain. **Cutting pains. Unbearable pain at the end of urination** – there may be no pain during urination. Terrible tenesmus **at the close of urination**.	Cutting and burning in the urethra **just after urination**. Urination whilst coughing, walking etc. Passes large quantities of urine. Clear mucus discharge from the urethra.	Irresistible urging to urinate in the daytime. Urinates after every drink. Burning and rawness. Stitching pains.	Sore cutting sharp pains. Dribbling of urine.
Site	**At the opening of the urethra**. In urethra.	Urethra, bladder.	Along urethra and **neck of bladder** (base of bladder where urethra joins).	
Modalities	< **At the end of urination**. During menses.	< **Just after finishing urinating**.	Urging < standing up.	
Urine	Offensive turbid urine. Often a dirty grey-green deposit. Pale, green. Sometimes bloody. Mucus and/or sediment – sandy urine. White sand with mucus, flaky urine.	Red sediment sometimes.	Normal colour and clear urine. If very cloudy then consider *Kali mur.* May be suppressed and scanty or excessive quantities.	**Thick, white mucus present**. Dark urine.
Concomitants	Inflammation of the kidneys especially if right sided – see *When to seek advice.*		If a cough is present this may cause the urine to spurt.	There may be associated pains in the kidneys – see *When to seek advice.* White or grey coating to the base of the tongue.
Peculiars				
Mentals and Generals (see texts)			Useful in the first stage of cystitis before there is any discharge or much cloudiness of the urine. It may be more commonly associated with people of a nervous, sensitive, pale disposition who may readily experience a flushing of the face.	Cystitis without specific characteristics of pain or urination but with thick, white mucus in the urine. It follows well after *Ferrum phos.* when the urine becomes cloudy.

Cystitis

Remedy	Kali phos.	Apis	Cantharis	Causticum
Cause & onset	From excitement, overwork or worry.		Rapid onset into a serious state.	From cold.
Sensations	Frequent urination or passes large quantities. Urine stops and starts. Incontinence from nervous debility – cannot hold urine from weakness of sphincter muscles. **Burning, scalding during urination** and continuing after. Cutting pains. Itching in the urethra.	Constant or frequent **desire to urinate** but only small amounts passed or even drops despite much straining. Must press to pass urine. Scanty urine. **Stinging pains.** Burning, pressing pains. Severe pains and urging. Last drops burn and smart.	**Burning during urination. Intolerable urging** and urgency to pass urine which may not be relieved after urination is complete. Urine may only be **passed in drops** with extreme pain. **Constant severe desire to urinate. Burning,** cutting and stabbing pains. **Severe pains.**	**Frequent desire to urinate** day and night but ineffectual – no urine passes or only a very little or has to wait a long time for little result and the desire returns soon after. Burning during urination. Sometimes will urinate a little when coughing, walking etc. or in sleep.
Site	**Bladder.** Sometimes in the urethra.	Bladder.	Bladder, bladder neck and urethra.	
Modalities	< During and after urination.	< **Heat.** At night. > Cold.	< Before, during and after urination. Cold drinks.	< During urination.
Urine	Yellow or milky.	**Scanty urine.** Bloody urine, foul.	**Bloody urine,** often very bloody.	May have sediments. Various colours, dark to light.
Concomitants	Bleeding from the urethra.	Thirstless. Abdomen very sensitive to touch. There may be **swelling** around the opening of the urethra. Inflammation in the kidneys – see *When to seek advice*.	Inflammation of the kidneys – see *When to seek advice*.	May have spasms in the rectum and constipation.
Peculiars				Itching at the orifice (opening) of the urethra.
Mentals and Generals (see texts)	Cystitis with marked weakness and prostration. Nervous weakness. For debilitated people, worn out and tremulous.	Especially if there is any swelling anywhere and the person is hot, wanting cool air and is better for it.	May double up and scream from the pains – a really **violent cystitis. Intensity and rapidity** mark this remedy. Great thirst. Uneasy, restless, distressed, wants to be moving about all the time.	

Cystitis

Remedy	Mag. phos.	Mercurius	Pulsatilla	Nux vomica
Cause & onset			From getting wet and cold, wet feet.	**Excesses** – of eating, alcohol, coffee etc.
Sensations	**Constant urging to urinate whenever standing or walking.** Spasm of the bladder, spasmodic retention of urine. Painful urging. **Cramping pains.** Shooting, burning pains on urinating. Cutting pains in the bladder before urinating.	**Uncontrollable urging** to urinate. **Constant desire, no llet up.** Urine passed in small amounts. Scanty urine passed very slowly. **Burning pains** especially if they are **worse when not urinating.**	**Cannot lie on the back without the desire to urinate. Great urgency.** Urging without effect. Has to concentrate on holding her urine. May pass urine in sleep. Urine only dribbles out – may dribble when coughs or sneezes etc. May be copious urine too. Smarting and burning. Pressure or cramp in bladder.	**Frequent,** urgent desire to urinate **but ineffectual, nothing comes.** Slight incontinence maybe. Burning or pressing pain in bladder during urination. Pain in urethra before or during urination. Itching in urethra and pain in neck of bladder whilst urinating.
Site	Bladder.	Urethra.		
Modalities		< **Night.** When not urinating or can be < before, at the start or at the end of urination.	Urging < **lying on back.**	< During urination. Cold and draughts.
	> Heat and pressure, bending double.	> Usually at the beginning of urination.		> Lying on back.
Urine	Gravel in the urine sometimes.	Dark urine, blood, mucus.	Bloody.	
Concomitants		Urine may be corrosive and cause itching and inflammation.		Urethral pain during urination with a strong urge to defecate.
Peculiars		Pains < when not urinating, > at beginning of urination.		
Mentals and Generals (see texts)			Touchy, weepy, changeable people. Hates heat and stuffiness. Thirstless etc.	Irritable, sensitive, nervous and chilly people etc.

Cystitis

Remedy	Staphisagria	Sulphur	Lycopodium	
Cause & onset	From suppressed emotions, indignation.			
Sensations	Frequent and painful urging to urinate. Involuntary urination. Burning during and after urination. May be > when urinating that is, only burns in urethra when **not** urinating.	Frequent desire with urgency especially at night. Incontinence at night. Sudden urge to go and must hurry but may only dribble or pass a few drops. **Burning** in urethra during urination and lasting a long time afterwards.	**Frequent urging to urinate** but ineffectual, **must wait a long time** before it passes, with a constant bearing down sensation – may support the abdomen with her hands. **Passes more urine at night than during the day.** Incontinence at night, in sleep. Dull, pressing and heaviness in bladder. Cutting stitching pains. Child may cry and toss around before urinating because she cannot and it hurts.	
Site	Urethra.	Urethra.		
Modalities	< Motion, walking etc. > When urinating sometimes.	< During urination. Frequency < at night.	> Riding in a car etc, that is, being rocked around.	
Urine	Bloody.	Like brown beer. Mucus or pus in urine. Smells foul.	Milky, turbid, bloody. Red sand in the urine.	
Concomitants	Acrid urine – may make the parts sore over which it flows.	Cystitis may follow a cold (coryza). Acrid urine – makes sore the parts over which it flows.	Renal colic – see *When to seek advice*. Problems with flatulence, feeling bloated after eating ever so little.	
Peculiars	Sensation as if a drop of urine is continuously rolling along the urethra, > when urinating.			
Mentals and Generals (see texts)	Indignation with trembling. The sense of being assaulted or of not having one's needs met at some incident prior to the cystitis may be a strong pointer to this remedy. Any sense of violation. Hence it may be a remedy for 'honeymoon cystitis' where the body can feel violated even if the woman does not. It may arise in sensitive, touchy people. Someone easily offended yet they do not express their inner anger etc.			

Cystitis: When to seek advice

Urgently, Right now!

- If there is a fever and inflammation of the kidneys. This causes pain in the kidney area (the loins). They lie on either side of the spine above the waist. If you place your hands on your hips with your fingers pointing backwards and then move them an inch or two higher over the bottom of the rib cage they will cover the loins.
- If there are rigors – bouts of cold and violent shivering and shaking.

Within 24 hours

- If any of the symptoms are severe.
- If there is a significant fever, above 101°F (38.4°C).
- If there is a significant amount of blood in the urine. It may be pink, red or a muddy-brown like tea (with milk in).
- If there is vomiting or a significant headache.
- If swelling of the hands, face or ankles develops.
- All males with cystitis should seek the advice of their health care practitioner, particularly if it is recurrent. It may be an indication of other problems in the urinary tract some of which could potentially be serious in the long term.

§12 Period pains

Whilst period pain may be helped each month by remedies selected from this table, the recurrent nature of these problems is unlikely to be affected until a more constitutional approach is adopted. See *Conditions Requiring Constitutional Therapy* on page 137.

In general, regular exercise helps to lessen period pains as may vigorous exercise during the painful time especially if it mobilises the pelvic area. If you practice Yoga, remember to avoid inverted postures during menstruation. Masturbation may help some people with particularly acute pains.

Period pains: When to seek advice

Urgently, Right now!

- If the pain is unusually severe.
- If a period has been missed and there is a possibility of pregnancy when severe or unusual pains develop with or without any blood flow.

Within 24 hours

- Significant bleeding between periods even without pains.
- Recurrent minor, unexplained bleeding between periods.
- Any uncharacteristic vaginal discharge, especially if accompanied by lower abdominal pain or fever.
- If sores develop on, in or near the genitals.
- If you have had sex with someone who is known to have a sexually transmissible disease like gonorrhoea, syphilis or chlamydia.

Period pains

Remedy	Mag. phos.	Colocynthis	Belladonna	Nux vomica
Sensations	Colicky, cramping pains **eased by curling up round a hot water bottle and pressing firmly**, often with a fist in the lower abdomen or firm pressure on the back.	Colicky, cramping pains **eased by steady pressure** and heat, very similar to *Mag. phos.* Sharp pains in the ovaries, especially if they precede the period.	Acute pains **begin and end suddenly. Violent** spasms of pain. Cramps or heavy, bearing down, pressure pains even as if everything would fall out of the pelvis (like *Sepia*). Sharp pains better bending backwards. There may be a sensation of heat in the pain.	Aching and cramping **pains in the lower back, in the sacrum**. May be accompanied by the desire to defecate even without a bowel movement. Pressing down pains extending into the rectum.
Radiation (where a pain moves to)	Pains can spread in all directions.	Cramps in the calf.		Pains in lower back (sacrum). Pains extending into the rectum.
Modalities	< Cold and draughts. > **Heat and firm pressure,** doubling up.	< Night. Suppressed anger. > **Steady pressure, doubling up** and heat.	< **Jar, walking, movement,** bending forward. Before and during menses. > Pressure (the bearing down pains). Straightening up or even bending backwards.	< **During the flow** – all symptoms. > Doubling up.
Menstrual flow			Bright red. Clotted. Heavy.	Profuse and long-lasting.
Concomitants	Clean tongue. Back ache > pressure and heat.	Coated tongue. Cramps in calf. Cramps may alternate with dizziness.	Ovarian pains before or during menses with typical *Belladonna* modalities – < jar, motion etc. Headache before and during menses. Red face, hot head, cold extremities may be present.	Constant but ineffectual desire to defecate or urge to urinate. Maybe constant nausea, even with faintness.
Peculiars				
Mentals and Generals (see texts)	Probably the most commonly required remedy for menstrual cramps. No mental symptoms with it of great note. If irritability is marked with demands for the pains to be relieved straight away this would favour *Colocynthis*.	Restless – rest drives her to despair. **Irritable** and angry unlike *Mag. phos.* Demands pain relief immediately. May hate to have anyone near them. Pains may follow or be made worse by anger, indignation, resentment or grief.	May be very sensitive, cannot have the body touched.	She may be very irritable, openly critical and fault finding. Not reserved with her anger. Can be very sensitive to light, noise, odours etc. Chilly too.

Period pains

Remedy	Conium	Pulsatilla	Chamomilla	Lachesis
Sensations	Stitching pains in breasts or nipples with swelling and tenderness to touch. Stitching pains in ovaries.	Any type of pain. Pains which vary from time to time and place to place.	**Cramps and bearing down pains.** Acute pains that may cause her to cry out. Unendurable pains.	Uterine cramps and soreness. Ovarian pains especially on the **left side.**
Radiation (where a pain moves to)	**Drawing down the thighs.**	Comes in different places.	Up and down inner thigh. From back to inner thigh.	To back, chest, upper abdomen.
Modalities		< Warm room. > Open air. Bending double.	< Night. Getting angry. > **Warmth**.	< Tight clothing around the waist. > **As soon as the flow begins – brings relief of all symptoms.**
Menstrual flow	May be scanty.	May be late or irregular, during the day only.	Dark blood. Profuse.	The less the flow the more the pain.
Concomitants	Heavy, swollen, lumpy breasts before menses, possibly extending to the flow as well. **Vertigo (dizziness)** < for turning the head.	Nausea, vomiting or diarrhoea. Fainting. Headache. Backache.	Hot flushed face and hot sweats with the cramps.	Back pain. Dizziness. Headache.
Peculiars				
Mentals and Generals (see texts)	**Exhaustion, weak and trembling** – palpitations even. Easily startled by noise.	Pains may cause person to cry out. Weepy, tearful, craving company and attention. Irritable but less than *Nux vomica*. See typical *Pulsatilla* picture in the *Materia Medica* texts. This may guide you to *Pulsatilla*.	**Markedly irritable and faultfinding.** Whining restlessness. Peevish. Impatient and intolerant of pain – very sensitive to pain. See typical *Chamomilla* picture in *Materia Medica* texts.	May be especially hot and needing fresh air at the time of the period.

Period pains

Remedy	Sepia	Cocculus	Cimicifuga	Calc. phos.
Sensations	**Dragging, pressing, bearing down pains. Pains like a ball**. Feels like all the insides will fall out – hence she sits with her legs crossed which helps. Dull, sore, bruised pains.	Cramps, griping pains. Colic, pressing pains. Uterine pains.	Menstrual cramps which **fly around all over the place. Dart from side to side.** Pains across pelvis from hip to hip. **Sharp** shooting pains.	Heavy, bearing down pains before and during menses.
Radiation (where a pain moves to)			**Low back pain** during menses.	Violent back ache.
Modalities	< **During menses**. Standing, walking, urinating. > Crossing legs, vigorous exercise.	< Movement – the motion of riding in a car. Breathing.	< Movement. During menses.	< From any change of weather. Pains < after stool or urination.
Menstrual flow	May be scanty.	Profuse, dark flow.	The more the flow, the more the pain. Profuse, dark, clotted. **Irregular menses**.	Late menses with violent backache. If late, blood is dark. Clotted. Heavy.
Concomitants		Bloated abdomen. Weakness. Piles.	Pains moving up or down the front of the thighs.	Rheumatic pains in joints. Pain with violent backache, vertigo, increased sexual desire or throbbing headache.
Peculiars	Sensations like a **ball or plug** in the affected part.		**Pains flying around.**	
Mentals and Generals (see texts)		May be very weak, utterly exhausted during the flow.	**Agitation and pain.** Great sensitivity and **intolerance to pain**.	Sexual desire increased before menses and great weakness and sinking after menses.

Period pains

Remedy	Ferrum phos.	Kali phos.	Calcarea fluorica	
Sensations	**Congested** feeling. Pressure in abdomen, small of back and top of head. Bearing down pains. Vagina dry, hot and sensitive.	Great pain with the flow. Colic, weight and fullness.	Excessive flow with bearing down pains in uterus and thighs.	
Radiation (where a pain moves to)	Constant, dull ovarian pains.	Pain across low back (sacrum).	Thighs.	
Modalities				
Menstrual flow	Bright red flow.	**Thin flow**, sometimes strong smelling. Irregular menses, early or late.	**Excessive flow, flooding.**	
Concomitants	Menses with **flushed face and a rapid pulse**. With vomiting of undigested food.	Dull headache with menses.	Hard, knotty lumps in breasts with or before menses.	
Peculiars	**Menses with a heavy pain on the top of the head (vertex).**			
Mentals and Generals (see texts)	If this congested, flushed pattern recurs every month then the remedy may be more effective if it is started a few days before the period is due.	Pale, weepy, irritable, sensitive ladies. Increased sexual desire after menses.	A remedy useful where there are problems of venous relaxation and congestion. Hence its value in varicose veins, piles etc.	

§13 Vaginal Thrush

This condition often arises when the system is out of balance. It may be connected with the use of drugs, especially antibiotics. The thrush organism, *Candida albicans*, is a yeast which is normally found on the skin. It only becomes a problem if the environment encourages it to grow excessively.

There are several general measures that can be taken to reduce or eliminate the problem altogether. Firstly try not to create the environment in which it grows well. It likes damp, moist, airless places with a slightly more alkaline pH than is normally found in the vagina (normally slightly acid). Therefore wear clothing that is loose and airy. Jeans, trousers and tights are much loved by *Candida*. Preferably wear a skirt or culottes with loose underwear made from natural fibres or better still no underwear at all. Rinse underwear thoroughly after washing. Some people find a change of soap powder can help, especially a move away from a biological powder. Also avoid the use of vaginal deodorants, tampons and bleached sanitary towels.

Soaps, bubble bath and the like are all alkaline and best avoided completely, especially the use of soap anywhere near the vagina. In fact, as a general comment on skin care, the less soap and detergent used the better. I frequently recommend that soap be used only if there is stubborn dirt that will not rub off without it. The problem is that soap washes out the natural skin oils which keep our skin supple and protect it from the ravages of the outside world. It is a myth, put about by parents and soap manufacturers, that we need soap in order to wash. Generally a good daily rub in the bath or shower is all that is required. You can actually feel that there is a grimy, slimy layer that disappears after a little rubbing leaving a soft slightly oily feel to the skin. Your skin needs those oils. If you wash them away it will either become dry and troublesome or the body will try to replace them and become too greasy. Apart from really dirty hands my family has not used soap for many years and our friends still come to visit us, even the blunt ones who are not slow to call a spade a spade!

Another factor which may initiate a bout of thrush is mechanical injury. If you make love when there is inadequate lubrication and you become dry, and/or sore, this can often encourage thrush. If this is a problem, be sure to use a good lubricant like KY Jelly (available at every chemist as far as I am aware). Thrush also arises as a means of unloading waste material from the body. It is a discharge of 'stuff' that the body cannot properly process. This may arise when there are excesses in the diet or when the digestive system is upset and weakened so that it cannot fully break down the food for the body to use. The latter is the case when antibiotics are taken which affect the natural balance of healthy organisms in the gut and thereby reduce its digestive capability for a while. Taking a little live yoghurt or a lactobacillus supplement (available as acidophilus capsules: the best are enteric coated, which prevent the capsule dissolving in the stomach where the acidophilus would be killed by the stomach juices thus allowing a safe passage to the lower gut where they are needed) will often help to restore this balance more quickly. Live yoghurt applied vaginally can often bring considerable relief from the itching, so long as you can contain the mess! Even more effective, I am told, is crushed garlic mixed with live yoghurt. It can also help on its own either locally or in the diet. *Excessive* quantities of dairy products, refined sugars and raw foods would be best avoided, with the emphasis on excessive. Part of the diet can be raw but not totally because raw foods require more digestive power than do cooked. If the digestion is already weakened then it will not cope with a totally raw food diet. As you may be able to see from the above, there are many factors that play a part in the condition called thrush. A constitutional assessment would be highly recommended particularly as thrush tends to be a recurrent or chronic problem – see *Conditions Requiring Constitutional Therapy* on page 137. However it is still worth trying one of the following remedies for an acute attack.

Kali mur. 6x. Probably the remedy to try first, two or three times a day especially if there is a thick, milky-white, bland discharge that does not irritate or only very little. The discharge may be quite profuse.

Sulphur 30. The itching is very troublesome and may be around the vagina with burning soreness and redness. It may be worse for any contact with water and when warm. Take a single dose of *Sulphur 30* but expect the thrush to get worse in three or four days' time before it will get better.

Pulsatilla 6x or 12. A burning, thick discharge like cream, especially if it occurs at the time of the monthly period. One, twice or three times daily. (See the *Materia Medica* for other *Pulsatilla* symptoms.)

Sepia 6x or 12. A milky discharge, if it is **lumpy**, in big lumps, then *Sepia* would be well worth trying. Even more so if there was dryness of the vagina and an aversion to sex. One, twice or three times a day. (See *Period Pains*.)

Candida 30. If all else fails try a single dose of *Candida 30*. (This remedy is unlikely to be available at your local stockists – see *Remedies and Pharmacies* on page 140).

§14 Birthing

It is of the greatest benefit if this process is approached with love and trust. Birthing is not something which you do with your mind. You do it with your body just like it has been successfully done millions of times before throughout history. Your body will perform regardless. It helps if your mind and emotions are in harmony with it and you have the loving support of those around you. Ideally, avoid the company of those who are afraid, even if they are trying not to show it. Spend as much time as possible with those who support you in every way. One of the best ways to achieve this harmony is through breathing. Practise breathing with the diaphragm, so that the tummy moves out and the bottom of the rib cage expands as you breath in, and vice versa as you breath out. The top of the chest should move very little. In early pregnancy you can practise this lying on your back with a bag of sugar or two on the upper part of your tummy. This helps to train the diaphragm to move. It will not be so easy later on! Practise breathing out fear and breathing in love and trust. All this will help your body to perform this creative function to the best of its ability.

Pregnancy is a wonderful time to have constitutional homoeopathic treatment because changes can happen much more quickly and simply than at other times resulting in a healthier more energetic body that will perform its functions with greater ease (see Chapter 1).

Preparations for pregnancy can begin six months or more before conception with a healthy diet – plenty of fresh fruit and vegetables, preferably organically grown and as few chemicals in the form of food additives as is possible. Also use as pure a source of water as possible for drinking and cooking. Stopping smoking and avoiding alcohol are also important. **All these measures apply to the man as well**. The quality of the sperm is important. Anyone interested in this aspect of preconceptual care would do well to contact Foresight who have local counsellors able to give specific individual advice. (See *Sources of Information*.)

The following remedies are intended to assist the body with some of the hold-ups that may occur in this natural process whether or not you are having constitutional treatment. Do not take them unless you need to and do not hesitate to use them if they are indicated. If the event does not live up to your expectations take whatever help and comfort you need from those willing to give it. Letting go of guilt and self-recrimination is not always easy. It may be comforting if you can acknowledge that in any moment you make the best choices you are able to in the situations in which you find yourself. With hindsight, it may not seem so. Better choices can usually be seen but can never be made retrospectively. A completely normal delivery is a rare event these days. It involves about twenty minutes of mild discomfort. I have only ever seen this once. Normality is rare in the 'civilised' Western world with regard to all aspects of health. However it can be achieved and is well worth pursuing.

The remedies in the 200M and 10M potencies will not be available over the counter except in specialist pharmacies. Suitable sources will be found in the section *Remedies and Pharmacies*.

Early labour

If the contractions cannot make up their mind about starting or not, that is they come and go and labour is not properly established, take one dose of *Pulsatilla 200* every 2 hours until the contractions do make up their mind. They will either stop or labour will start properly. In either case take no more.

Established labour

Once the process is definitely under way and there is no chance of it stopping again take **one dose only** of *Caulophyllum 10M*.

Exhaustion

The process is becoming laborious and a lot of energy is being expended with little result to show for it, progress is very slow. The nervous system is becoming exhausted. Take one dose of *Kali phos. 12x* every 15 minutes until the results justify the effort being made.

Lack of trust, fear

If the mother or anyone else connected with the birthing process shows any signs of lack of trust, anxiety, fear, pain, etc. take one dose as often as needed, perhaps as often as every 10 minutes, of *Rescue Remedy* (one of the Bach Flower remedies). It is available as pills or as a liquid and can if wanted be put in a glass of water to be sipped.

The baby at birth

Ideally, the cord should be allowed to stop pulsating before it is clipped or cut. Be prepared to express your preference to your attendants. If the new person shows any signs of shock or fright, or if he or she stays purple for too long then give one dose of *Aconite M*. If the baby is still attached by the cord to the mother then she may take it. It would be best to buy this remedy as liquid potency for ease of administration. If this is not possible you can crush a pill between two spoons to make a powder which can be sprinkled onto the lips and tongue of the baby if needed. Prepare this remedy before labour starts.

Bleeding

If there is any sign of overbleeding after the arrival of the new person give one dose of *Ipecacuanha 200*. Take one dose only. Any bleeding should stop in seconds or a minute or two. The brisker the bleeding the quicker it should stop.

Immediately after the birth

Give the new mother one dose of *Arnica 200* every 3 hours for **three doses only**. Start as soon as the delivery is complete. It will help the body to quickly recover from any stretching, bruising or damage that it may have sustained.

The next day

Take one dose of *Bellis perennis M.* each day for three days starting the day after the birth. It will help the mother's organs to regain their natural places.

§15 Breast feeding

You need to be comfortable and the baby needs to be well supported. Pillows may be useful. Breast feeding lying down is restful, especially at night and for an afternoon nap. Make sure that the baby's body is facing the breast and that he or she is taking the whole nipple to fill its mouth. The best description I have heard for this position is 'well plugged on' – a plug will not go into a socket if it is crooked, that is the baby should not be twisting his or her neck. Try looking over your shoulder and drinking a glass of milk. Many babies also find this position uncomfortable and will, not surpisingly, prefer the bottle. If you are having problems you could get in touch with an experienced breast feeding counsellor from one of the self-help organisations. Here are a few remedies to help with some of the more commonly encountered problems during breast feeding.

Cracked and sore nipples

Keep the nipples dry and exposed to the air; pads can make things worse.

Castor equi 3x. Sore nipples, cracked and ragged, exceedingly sensitive, cannot bear touch. The number one remedy.

Phytolacca 6x or 12. Sore and fissured. Retracted nipples. Pain starts in the nipple and radiates all over the body. Intense pains. May have heavy breasts with hard lumps.

Hydrastis 6x or 12. Abrasions (grazes) of the nipple. Retracted nipples.

Mastitis

This is inflammation and infection of the breast which sometimes follows cracked nipples and shows itself by pain, redness of a part or the whole breast, swelling, and fever. If you are feeling 'fluey' this may be the first sign of mastitis. You should consult your health care practitioner if you suspect that mastitis is on the way but start with the following measures immediately.

It is important to keep on breast feeding and to empty, as far as possible, the affected breast. This will help the breast to clear the infection and may in itself prevent a mild bout from getting worse. **It will not harm your baby**. You will be producing antibodies in your milk which will protect him or her. In order to empty the breast completely it is best to feed with the baby in one of three different positions:

1. Cradling the baby in front of you in the traditional way, see above.

2. with the baby under your arm, like a rugby or an American football player carrying a ball whilst running.
3. Whilst lying down with the baby beside you in line with your body.

These positions will help the breast to drain from all its segments. Cold or hot compresses and/or a gentle massage may bring some relief.

In the early stages of inflammation one of the first three remedies will probably be indicated. The first two are the most commonly required. Remedies will not hurt the baby.

Bryonia. Inflammation due to consolidation of milk. Worse (<) **Movement – must** support the breast. Pains may be stitching, tearing.

Belladonna. Bright **red** and very **hot**. A segment of the breast affected, streaks of red. Rapid onset. Frightfully tender. Burning, **throbbing** pains. Worse (<) **jar**, least touch.

Mercurius. When *Bryonia* and *Belladonna* fail! Worse (<) Heat, cold, everything. Not even relieved by sweating. Ulcerating pains.

Phytolacca. When the breast becomes hard, like stone with great pain. Painful, very hard lumps, especially if associated with an injury, either recent or in the past. When suppuration becomes inevitable (an abscess is forming).

Hepar sulphuris. After suppuration has begun when there is intense heat and throbbing.

See also the *Fever* sections and the *Materia Medica* for more information.

Milk supply

Pulsatilla. Given immediately upon stopping the nursing this will often help to dry up the milk supply.

Calcarea carbonica or *Lac defloratum.* May help to increase an inadequate milk supply. Ideally an assessment by an experienced practitioner should be sought for this but these two remedies are worth trying.

After pains during breast feeding

Arnica. May help especially if it has not already been given directly after the birth. Violent pains.

Conium. Pains which go from left to right.

Post-natal depression

Post-natal depression or prolonged 'blues' really needs assessment by an experienced practitioner. See *Conditions Requiring Constitutional Therapy*' on page 137.

§16 Baby colic

Here are four of the most commonly indicated remedies with their key symptoms. A more detailed description plus a comparison with other colic remedies will be found in the *Abdominal Complaints* tables.

Mag. phos. Better (>) **heat**, doubling up, firm pressure. Passing wind or belching may not help. Persistent hiccup with retching may occur. The number one remedy for colics.

Colocynthis. Better (>) **pressure**, heat, doubling up. More restless, irritable and angry than *Mag. phos.* The tongue may also be coated. Pressure relieves more in *Colocynthis* and heat in *Mag. phos.* Otherwise they are very similar.

Chamomilla. Doubles up and **screams** with a hot, flushed face and sweat. **Frantically irritable**. The inconsolable temper will often indicate this remedy.
Better (>) heat, being carried.
Worse (<) at night.
There may also be green diarrhoea and a smell of rotten eggs.

Dioscorea. Worse (<) doubling up.
Better (>) stretching out, heat and firm pressure.
The colic may be very sudden. Better (>) stretching out is the key to this remedy.

§17 Teething and toothache

Chamomilla. Irritable, piteous wailing, even a snarling cry. Nothing suits; capricious desires, wants this, no, that! Whenever a thing demanded is offered it is rejected. Does not know what he wants. One gets exasperated with the *Chamomilla* child, unlike the *Pulsatilla* child who most often evokes one's sympathy. The only relief is from being constantly carried and even then the relief may not last or they will want to be carried first by one parent and then the other. A hot head. Aching, tearing, stitching, burning pains.

Worse (<) night; warm food or drinks; warm room or bed.
Better (>) cold drinks held in the mouth, cold air.

Pulsatilla. Very weepy, whiny and clingy. They desire company and to be held and touched. There may be tearing and stitching pains.

Worse (<) warm drinks; lying with the head low.
Better (>) cold water held in the mouth; cold air; walking in the open air; pressure.

Bryonia. Tearing stitching pains.

Worse (<) warmth; motion; smoking.
Better (>) cold drinks held in the mouth; cold air; firm pressure.

Mercurius. Salivation. Offensive odour of mouth is marked. Sweetish or metallic taste. There may be perspiration with it. Drawing pain.

Worse (<) cold air; cold drinks; smoking.
Characteristically things tend to aggravate (<) and nothing ameliorates (>).

Coffea. In a nervous person, grinds teeth. Hasty eating and drinking.

Worse (<) hot food and warm drinks.
Temporarily better (>) by holding cold water in the mouth; biting teeth together; eating.

Calc. phos. Slow dentition or early decay. Foul taste, bitter. Coated, swollen tongue. Sensitive to touch, pressure, chewing.

Worse (<) cold; cold air on teeth.

Ignatia. Teeth feel numb. Toothache on waking. Bites inside of cheek when chewing.

Worse (<) after drinking tea, coffee, wine; smoking.
Better (>) pressure; biting teeth together.

Kreosotum. Rapid decay, crumbling teeth with spongy bleeding gums. Putrid odour and bitter taste. Pains radiate to the ear or temples.

The pain of a tooth abscess or following extraction may be relieved by a solution of *Hypericum* and *Calendula* (or *Calendula* alone) as a mouthwash, using two teaspoons full of the tincture in half a glass of water.

§18 Measles

Aconite. **Sudden onset** of fever; restlessness; restless sleep; nasal discharge is clear; red eyes; photophobia; dry croupy cough with stitches in the chest. Only of use early in the illness when there is suddenness and violence. Thirst; itching burning skin; restless; tossing; anxious and fearful.

Belladonna. Sudden onset again, with a **burning red skin**; high fever; dryness and usually thirst; throbbing headache; drowsy and may be delirious; cannot sleep; twitches and jerks; starts and jumps; sore throat; swollen face; hot head and cold extremities.
Worse (<) light – cannot bear it, noise, pressure or jar.
Better (>) heat.

Ferrum phos. In the early stages if no other remedy is clearly indicated or if *Aconite* seems to be indicated but does not help at all.

Apis. High fever; **oedema** and highly inflamed eyes and lips; thirstless; may be tearful irritable and delirious. Especially when the rash does not come out or is suppressed and a stuporose state comes on; stinging pains; high pitched cry; scanty urine; swellings and effusions.
Worse (<) heat and better (>) cool – in any form.

Bryonia. Sore limbs and body; child wants to lie **still and not be moved**; any movement and the child may scream with pain; dry mouth and mucus membranes; intense **thirst for cold water**; a bitter taste in the mouth, food or drink. When the rash appears late or the chest is particularly affected; dry, hard, painful cough with chest stitches or tearing pains; twitches of muscles; pale face; eyes red; constipation and frequently **frontal headaches**; mild delirium and the child 'wants to go home'.
Worse (<) motion.
Better(>) cold and still.

Euphrasia. Measles rash and fever with **fluent bland coryza and acrid watery or purulent eye discharge**; inflammation round the eye; eyes appear red and bright; streaming, hot, burning tears with the rash; photophobia; intense, throbbing, headache which is better (>) once the rash appears; dry cough. Nose and eyes better (>) open air.

Pulsatilla. If there is very high fever then *Pulsatilla* is not likely to be indicated. It is frequently required in measles.
Very **weepy and clingy**; erratic temperature and **changeable symptoms; thirstless**; often accompanied by some sort of digestive upset – nausea or diarrhoea after the fever has passed; chilly but **dislikes the heat; thick, yellow,**

bland discharges; earache; lingering eye complaints; dry cough at night and loose by day; **desires cool open air**. (Consider *Kali bich.* too.)

Gelsemium. **Slow onset**; gradual fever and chilliness which may run up and down the back; feels very **heavy and tired**, so he is motionless, apathetic, drowsy, dislikes disturbances; thirstless; watery coryza which burns the upper lip; **occipital dull heavy headache**; sometimes a harsh croupy cough; chills and heats chase each other; sneezing; sore throat; face dark red, swollen with a besotted look; ptosis; **so tired, weak and feels stupid**.

Rhus tox. **Great soreness and restlessness**; stupor and mild delirium – child constantly tossing about; very itchy rashes not relieved by scratching; rash is also dry, hot and burning; desire cold drinks.

Worse (<) at rest; at night.

Kali bich. This remedy may come in later if earache occurs; enlarged lymph glands; sensation of pressure at the root of the nose or throbbing and burning; rattling cough; thick, yellow, stringy nasal discharge.

Camphor. When the rash fails to appear; child is **very cold yet wants to kick off the covers; desires fresh air**; rather pinched face; may have profuse diarrhoea.

Sulphur. The rash **stings and burns, is worse (<) washing and water, worse (<) heat of the bed**; thirsty; hot feet, may stick them out of the bed; hot flushes of the skin which may look dusky and red; burning stinging catarrhs from the eyes or nose; dusky purplish skin and the rash does not come out; **slow convalescence and the patient is weak, tired and prostrate**.

Mercurius. Catarrhal measles with abundant rash and earache; thick, swollen, heavily coated tongue; offensive breath; swollen, ulcerated eyelids; often loose motions.

Carbo veg. Congestive headache; dusky face; enlarged lymph glands, even induration; alternating heat and chill; warm head and cold extremities; wants to be fanned vigorously.

Arsenicum. Severe measles; **great restlessness; prostration; anxiety; offensive and exhausting discharges, diarrhoea; delirium**.

See also *Fevers* and any other sections as appropriate.

§19 Mumps

Belladonna. **Rapid onset and violent**. Dazed and delirious with twitchings and startings; **high fever; great redness**, red face, swelling, inflammation, heat of parotids worse (<) touch. Dryness; burning in the throat; shooting pains in glands; **throbbing** headache; spasms in the throat with difficulty swallowing; often a copious thirst but may be thirstless; **dilated pupils; hot head** and cold extremities; wants heat; fine smooth rash. Child may wet the bed and have constipation. Especially affects the right side.

Phytolacca. Swollen, inflamed parotids; submandibular glands too – they may be stony hard with a sensation of tension or pressure around them; pains often **shoot into the ears on swallowing**; dry rough throat with difficulty swallowing especially hot things; pale face and skin. Generally worse (<) cold and wet weather, at night, the heat of the bed. May be needed when the swelling subsides as the result of a chill and worse ensues, such as the breast, ovaries or testicles becoming affected.

Jaborandi. Dry mouth with copious salivation, saliva like the white of an egg; intense thirst; enlarged submaxillary glands; dry at the back of the throat; furred tongue and difficulty talking; swelling of the tonsils and stiffness of the jaws; profuse sweat. When swelling subsides as the result of a chill and worse ensues, like *Phytolacca*, when it affects the breasts, ovaries or testes.

Mercurius. Profuse **sweat and salivation** with a **foul odour; sweating** worse at night; **offensive**; foul metallic, sweet taste; enlarged submandibular glands; swollen tongue showing indents from the teeth; glands may be hard and tender; right side especially. Use in the later stages after the fever.

Pulsatilla. In the later stages if it lingers, with a **weepy clingy** child **desiring open air** and is **worse in a warm room; thirstless**; heavily coated tongue – yellow or white; dry mouth; bad taste; enlarged glands everywhere. Worse (<) night, lying down; **inflammation extends to the breasts or testes.**

Apis. Red, oedematous **swelling; burning and stinging pains; face puffed and pitted**; swollen eyelids; cannot bear to be left alone; very sensitive to touch or pressure; sweat comes and goes. **Worse (<) heat**. Like *Pulsatilla*, wants the covers off and cool things.

Aconite. If there is **very sudden onset of fever, great restlessness and thirst**; worse (<) warm room; better (>) open air.

Rhus tox. Swelling more on **left** than right; aching sore limbs, worse at night with restlessness; extreme chilliness and **sensitivity to the cold**; dry burning thirst; cold sores on the lips; highly inflamed and enlarged parotid and submaxillary glands, **worse (<) cold, cold winds, cold wet.**

Bryonia. Very **irritable and wants to be left alone**; slightest **motion causes pain**, even turning the head; dry lips and copious **thirst for cold water**.

Arsenicum. Severe weakness, **chilliness**, clammy sweats, **anxiety and thirst for sips**; also has extension of the illness to the breasts, ovaries and testes; worse after midnight.

Carbo veg. Face pale and cold; there may be a cold sweat on the forehead; breasts and testes may be involved.

Lachesis. Enormously **swollen parotid especially on the left side**; sensitive to the least **touch or pressure** which causes severe pain, he shrinks away when approached; can scarcely swallow, throat sore internally; face red and swollen; eyes glassy and wild. There is not the offensive mouth and dirty tongue of *Mercurius* but there is more **throbbing** with the *Lachesis* tension, like a pot on the boil, a sense of pent up energy.

Lycopodium. From **right to left side**; desires warm drinks which ameliorate (>); no offensive mouth and salivation of *Mercurius*.

See also *Fevers* and any other sections as appropriate.

§20 Chicken pox

Rhus tox. Intense itching worse (<) scratching, night and rest. May have large and pus filled eruptions; very **restless** and great difficulty going to sleep.

Pulsatilla. **Weepy clingy** children; worse (<) **heat**; little thirst despite the fever and dryness; better (>) **open air**; worse (<) night. Enlarged lymph nodes; light sweat and **low fever**; can be itchy when warm.

Ant. tart. Skin rash coming out very slowly and possibly a very large rash; may have a rattling cough and bronchitis. Pustular or blue rash with a cold skin sometimes. Child does not like to be touched or even looked at; **very ill humoured**; moans, whines and complains; often a white tongue, thickly coated; white sputum; nausea and gagging.

Arsenicum. Large eruptions with much pus – they may even become open sores like in *Mercurius*; **burning** pains better (>) **heat** or **hot applications** is very characteristic of this remedy; extreme **chilliness**; pain and itching worse (<) after midnight and worse (<) cold.

Belladonna. With severe headache, **red flushed face, very hot skin**, drowsy and unable to sleep, twitchings and startings etc.

Mercurius. With **offensive sweat**, profuse sweat. Large eruptions with much pus that may become open sores like *Arsenicum*. **Swollen glands** in the neck; never comfortable because they are worse (<) both by heat and cold, at night too. The discharges irritate and make the skin sore; salivation may be profuse; the breath offensive. Vesicles that suppurate. This remedy picture emerges more commonly after the fever.

See also *Fevers* and any other sections as appropriate.

Cocculus. Sick headache. Feels faint, empty and weak all over as if he would sink away; a sensation of hollowness as if the parts had gone to sleep, an emptiness and he **must lie down**. Averse to food. Feels too weak to talk. Dizziness, nausea and vomiting all worse (<) getting up. Waves of nausea.

Worse (<) cold; after eating; fresh air; movement.
Better (>) lying down.

Petroleum. An empty, **hungry feeling** or a pain in the stomach that makes him want to eat. Occipital headache with nausea, with vertigo, **or dizziness**. Excessive salivation. Worse (<) **fresh air**.

Sepia. Nausea with a feeling of emptiness or **sinking in the stomach**. Nausea with a headache which is worse (<) bending down or moving about. Sour belching or vomiting of bile.

Worse (<) thinking about food; eating; mornings.
Better (>) fresh air, especially the headache.

Staphisagria. May help for nausea in someone who is very indignant and 'uptight' that it should be happening to them. Sensitive and offended.

Tabacum. Much nausea, great pallor. A cold body, profuse cold sweat and exhaustion. Dizziness may be worse (<) in fresh air though it ameliorates (>) the nausea.

Worse (<) warmth, movement, stuffy room.
Better (>) open **air**; fanning; quiet and dark; closing eyes.

See also *Nux vomica* as a further possibility (*Materia Medica* section).

Note: The Chinese have used *Ginger* (stem or root) for nausea for over 2000 years. In its crystallised form or as ginger biscuits it may also help.

PART 3

First Aid Remedies

The suggestions for when to seek advice in the following sections are only intended to be guidelines to help you decide when you need to call on the expert help of your health care practitioner. Clearly your own knowledge, experience and circumstances will all play a part in your decision. The following guides do not aim to be totally comprehensive. Complete books have been written on this subject which will give much more information about when a condition is likely to be serious or not. For this reason the guidelines here tend to err on the cautious side.

§22 Index to first aid remedies

- The most important remedies are shown in **bold**.
- For emergency advice see page 103

Bites and stings	Apis, **Led., Nat. m.**, Staph, Urt. u.
Bruises	**Arn.**, Bellis., Hyper., Lach., Led., Ruta., Symph.
Burns	Cal., Canth., Caust., Phos., Urt. u.
Cuts and Scrapes	**Cal.**, Hyper., Staph.
Dislocated joints	**Arn.**, Ruta.
Eye trauma	**Euphr.**, Lach., **Symph**.
Fractures	Arn., Bry., Calc. p, Eup. per., Sil., **Symph**.
Head injuries	Arn., Kali. phos., Nat. sul.
Heat exhaustion	**Bell.**, Cupr., **Glon**.
Puncture wounds	Apis, Hyper., **Led**.
Sepsis	Lach.
Shock	**Arn**.
Strains and sprains	**Arn.**, Bellis., Bry., Calc. p., Led., **Rhus. t**, Ruta.

Bites and stings

Apis. Marked redness, swelling, heat and pain. Pains worse (<) heat. Often needed in urticaria (nettlerash) which develops after a bite or sting (see *Urtica urens* also).

Ledum. Number one remedy for bee stings. Swelling, redness, stinging and pricking pains. Part feels cold, yet is ameliorated (>) by cold applications.

Natrum mur. Very good remedy for bee and wasp stings. The remedy can even be made into a paste and applied directly to the sting.

Staphisagria. Especially in children who get mosquito bites which become large and irritating.

Urtica urens. For people with hives (nettle rash or urticaria) after a sting.

A.L.C. tincture can be applied to all sorts of stings and bites. It is a combination of *Apis*, *Ledum* and *Calendula*.

Bruises

Arnica. Anywhere. The number one remedy. Sore, bruised, aching.

Bellis per. For deep injuries to muscles and joints when *Arnica* does not seem to be working well enough.

Hypericum. Severe. Crushed parts, especially sentient parts (see *Cuts and Scrapes*), with the same excruciating, shooting pains and great sensitivity to touch. Pain like this after a fall on the coccyx. Spinal concussion.

Lachesis. Black eyes. Aids blood reabsorbtion. Worse (<) heat, better (>) cold, as above.

Ledum. Black eyes or severe bruises. Bruises that feel cold and numb. **Cold to touch and** better (>) **cold**, cold applications.

Ruta. Bruises of the periosteum of bones (it lies on the surface of bones and is easily injured where the bones lie just beneath the skin, for example, elbow, shin or kneecap). Sore, bruised, lame feelings.

Symphytum. In trauma to a cartilage or periosteum (the lining of a bone) especially near to the skin where pain is excessive and *Ruta* has not relieved within 24 hours. Blunt injury to the eyeball.

Burns

Calendula. For redness without blistering, that is, first degree burns, it is the number one remedy. It is also used to dress second degree burns (blisters without skin loss) once the blisters have broken leaving an open sore (see *Cuts and Scrapes*).

Cantharis. For blistering burns, that is, second degree, it is the number one remedy. After the blisters have broken dress locally with *Calendula* tincture.

Causticum. The number one remedy in third degree burns, that is, the full thickness of the skin has been lost. These are serious burns requiring medical attention and often skin grafting. Also of use in old burns that do not resolve and if there are any ill effects of burns – other conditions that have developed from the burn itself or coincided with the burn though not apparently directly connected with it.

Phosphorus. Electrical burns or shocks.

Urtica urens. Minor burns without blistering (first degree).

Other preparations recommended for minor burns include *Nelson's Burn Ointment* and *Pakua*, a wonderful preparation which aids healing in all sorts of injuries where the skin is damaged. (See *Sources of Information*.)

Cuts & Scrapes

Calendula. Use the tincture topically in a dilution of 1:25 with sterile or boiled water instead of an antiseptic to clean and dress shallow wounds. Excessive pain. In clean cuts with stinging pains. Torn lacerations. As a mouthwash after dental extraction. Treats and prevents suppuration. (Obtain and use *Calendula cerate* or ointment in episiotomies where it is very soothing.) **Do not use if deep sepsis is present** because it promotes rapid healing which will seal the sepsis (infection) in.

Hypericum. Use in deep cuts with much pain and hypersensitivity to any touch. Lacerated fingers. Use in injury to sentient parts – fingers, toes, anus, spine, coccyx, palms, soles, teeth. Pains characteristically shoot from the site of injury and often there is great stiffness. Excruciating pain, intolerable, shooting.

Staphisagria. In **clean cuts**. Injuries from **sharp instruments** with stinging and smarting. Lacerations, use after operations. Worse (<) **motion**, better (>) heat and better (>) pressure.

Dislocated joints

Arnica. The number one remedy. May need *Rhus tox.* or another remedy to follow after the joint has been reduced (put back in place).

Ruta. For repeated easy dislocation of joints after they have been relocated.

Eye trauma

Euphrasia. For the ill effects of bruises and other mechanical trauma, after *Arnica.* Conjunctivitis after injury; the eyes are hot, burning and watering. Soreness. Generally feels better in the open air, except the eyes which stream. It can also be most soothing when used in an eyebath. Sterile eye drops can be purchased for this purpose.

Lachesis. Black eyes. Aids blood reabsorbtion. Worse (<) heat, better (>) cold, as above.

Symphytum. Blunt injury to the eyeball such as when a tennis or squash ball hits the eye.

Fractures

Arnica. Helps with the shock, bruising and swelling. Often the first remedy needed because of the shock, which is the main indication. Local area very tender.

Bryonia. Sometimes in fractured ribs with marked worse (<) movement, must keep absolutely still and may even lie on the affected side in order to keep it from moving.

Calc. phos. Aids the nutrition of bones. May be of use if someone is malnourished or the bones are not healing (non-union).

Eupator. perf. Main symptom is pain without so much bruising as would make one give *Arnica.*

Silica. May be of use if a small chip has come off a bone.

Symphytum. The number one remedy. **Use only after the bones have been set.** Also may be of use in cases of non-union of a fracture. *Calc. phos.* may be needed after it. Irritating, pricking, stitching sharp pain in the point of the fracture.

Head injuries

Please take special note of the section at the end of this chapter on when to seek advice.

Arnica. For the shock and/or the bruising – the number one remedy.

Kali phos. When there is weakness and exhaustion after a head injury.

Natrum sul. With a headache, especially a crushing, gnawing pain in the occiput. Drowsiness, photophobia, buzzing or pain in the top of the head (vertex). (*Note.* Medical advice should be sought for such injuries with drowsiness or photophobia.) Better (>) cold air. This remedy may come in if there are any ill effects after a head injury, even as far as a change in personality but expert assistance should be sought in such cases.

Sun/heat stroke

Belladonna. Fever. Throbbing headache, bright-red face, stupor. Burning of the skin greater than with *Glonoin*. Headache better (>) bending the head backwards, better (>) sitting silently, better (>) head uncovered.

Cuprum. **Heat exhaustion. Cramping** marks out this remedy. Stupor with jerking of muscles and even convulsions may occur. Profuse, clammy sweat; great weakness even to collapse. Faintness, pallor, coldness of the body, nausea, a rapid pulse.

Glonoin. **Sunstroke** fever, throbbing headache, red face, stupor. Less burning of the skin than in *Belladonna* and worse (<) bending head backwards, worse (<) cold applications, better (>) uncovering and in the open air, better (>) pressure.

Puncture wounds

Apis. They feel warm or hot with stinging pains and better (>) cold applications. Much swelling at the site.

Hypericum. With the same excruciating, intolerable shooting pains in sentient parts (see *Cuts and Scrapes*).

Ledum. Number one remedy. Redness, swelling and throbbing pains. When the wound feels cold to touch but is better (>) by cold applications.

Sepsis

Lachesis. Suppuration (pus formation) after injury, sloughing, haemorrhage. This remedy has an affinity for the blood and circulation. Bad effects of poisoned wounds. An incredible sepsis remedy. Skin cold and clammy. Worse (<) heated room, better (>) touch. Better (>) cold air or being slowly fanned, better (>) once discharge has started.

Shock

Arnica. The number one remedy. Usually is the first remedy needed in any accident or injury.

Sprains and strains

Arnica. Muscles, ligaments or joints. After overexertion of muscles; pulled muscles with pain and stiffness; number one remedy for muscles. After overexertion or straining of ligaments and joints when there is considerable swelling, bruising and inflammation around the joint. Often *Rhus tox.* or another remedy is needed to follow before complete resolution occurs.

Bellis per. With deep injuries to muscles and joints when *Arnica* does not seem to be working well enough.

Bryonia. Ligament and joints. When the pain is worse (<) for the slightest movement and continued motion only makes it worse still. Some swelling.

Calc. phos. Where nutrition is a problem causing healing to be slow and prolonged. It may be used to supplement the action of the indicated remedy in such anaemic or malnourished people.

Ledum. Affecting fibrous tissues and joints, especially of ankles when parts feel cold or numb and are better (>) cold applications.

Rhus tox. Ligaments and muscles. Of muscles due to overexertion, after the most acute symptoms have gone or when there is worse (<) initial motion and better (>) from continued motion with better (>) heat. Of ligaments and joints where it is the number one remedy. Pains and stiffness are worse (<) initial motion, better (>) continued motion and better (>) heat. For complaints coming on after overexertion or over lifting. It often follows the initial use of *Arnica* in strains.

Ruta. Of ligaments and tendons. Usually of use after the most marked initial swelling and tenderness has begun to decline. In cases that do not have a clear *Rhus tox.* picture. Sore lame and bruised. Paralytic rigidness as if broken.

A few general notes about some of the remedies

Arnica. Use in bruises and shock. The sore, bruised, aching feeling makes him restless; always having to change position. Worse (<) touch; does not want anyone to come near him. He may say he is all right when he is not. In severe injury or in head injury he may lapse in and out of unconsciousness. It should be plain that cases such as this require urgent, expert medical attention for which *Arnica* is no substitute even though it may well help.

Calendula. Has an affinity with soft tissue conditions. **Excessive pain** is most characteristic. It helps clot formation and keeps a wound clean.

Ledum. Generally chilly and cold but they desire the cold. This remedy has an affinity for fibrous tissues, joints and tendons.

Rhus tox. The grand characteristics of this remedy are the **worse (<) from first movement and better (>) for continued movement with better (>) heat and worse (<) cold**. It has a strong affinity for fibrous tissues hence its use in conditions affecting joints, ligaments and the stage of healing when fibrous scar tissue is laid down after the initial inflammation has begun to settle.

When to seek advice

Urgently, Right now!

- In bites and stings if the creature is known to be poisonous or the person is known to react badly to such bites or stings.
- If after a bite or sting the conscious level is impaired or if swelling is severe and rapid especially if it affects the mouth and throat or if breathing becomes difficult.
- In burns – any third degree burn (see below), any second degree burn (blistering and loss of the top surface of the skin – very sore and painful) occurring on sensitive skin (face, hands, genitals) or second degree burn larger than a hand size occurring anywhere else. In electrical burns remember to isolate the power before touching the person, otherwise pull them off using some insulating material such as rubber, plastic or dry wood. Third degree burns involve the full thickness of the skin and are likely to be less tender than first or second degree burns so do not be fooled into underestimating the severity of a serious burn by the lack of pain. Do not dress or interfere with severe burns until expert help is available but do treat the shock. Other remedies may be needed later.
- If there is loss or impairment of consciousness or confusion after any form of trauma.
- Head injuries followed by:-
  1. Any impairment of consciousness from being drowsy and lethargic to total unconsciousness.
  2. Unexpected irritability.
  3. Any sign of neurological (nervous system) disturbance, such as slurred speech, visual abnormality (double, blurred, etc.), weakness or difficulty when moving the limbs, pupils of different size, numbness, fits or convulsions.
  4. Vomiting.
  5. Loss of a clear or a bloodstained, watery fluid from the nose or ear.
- If a fracture or serious neck or back injury is suspected. Do not move the person until expert help is available.
- Any joint injury with loss of the full range of movement of the joint, albeit painful!
- If the injured part is distorted, deformed or unstable in any way.
- Intense pain or spasm of the surrounding muscles which may suggest a fracture.
- If there is marked swelling or bleeding under the skin.
- Coldness, blueness, or numbness of the injury, or the part beyond the injury, suggesting damage to the blood or nervous supply of that area.
- In heat exhaustion (when the person has the symptoms of mild shock – cold, clammy, pale, tired, nausea, raised heart rate, they may also have muscle

cramps) if the level of consciousness is affected (drowsy and dull) or they do not show signs of increasing strength and vitality after an hour of cool rest.

- In sunstroke. This is a medical emergency because the body's temperature regulating mechanism has been overloaded and has failed. The skin is hot, red and often dry. There are signs of impaired consciousness or confusion and even convulsions. Take whatever steps are possible to cool the body below 102°F (38.9°C) as quickly as possible whilst awaiting expert help.
- Haemorrhage (bleeding). Obviously the severity of the wound and the bleeding will dictate the degree of urgency and need for help.
- Deep puncture wounds or animal bites anywhere.
- Lacerations and puncture wounds to the following areas should be treated with great caution as there are vital organs, blood vessels and nerves close to the surface – the face, neck, chest, abdomen, and back.
- If a wound appears to involve a joint, most commonly the knee.
- For signs of shock – pale, sweaty, faint or weak with cold limbs and a rapid, weak pulse.

Within 24 hours

- If a wound becomes infected as shown by increasing pain, swelling and redness, particularly if the inflammation runs from the wound in red streaks towards the body (lymphangitis). There may be suppuration.
- All animal bites should be examined by your health practitioner. His advice should also be sought for all puncture wounds and lacerations regarding any measures needed to avoid tetanus.
- Any unexpected impairment of use of the injured part, such as being unable to weight-bear on an injured leg or limited and painful use of a wrist after a fall, especially in a child.

Refer to other chapters as necessary.

PART 4

Materia Medica

Aconite

- Suddenness and intensity
- Exposure to cold, especially very cold dry weather and then ill the same day
- Great excitement of the circulation
- Fear
- Awful anxiety, anguish, great restlessness
- Oversensitive and burning pains
- Great thirst for cold water
- Bright red in its inflammations

Suddenness and intensity mark out *Aconite*. A great storm that suddenly appears and is soon over; if the condition lingers or does not have much intensity, it is not *Aconite*. *Aconite* is not feeble!

Often found to be needed in vigorous, robust, healthy, rugged people and in children: they come down suddenly with a violent illness, a raging fever etc. It has often been precipitated by a period of considerable **exposure to cold, especially very cold dry weather and then ill the same day**, that is soon after the exposure. It can also come in for gastric complaints following intensely hot weather. Illnesses may follow a fright or shock especially in children.

There is **great excitement of the circulation**; a full, fast pulse; great nervousness and excitement without much delirium. In the extreme this can lead to intense **fear**, even to predicting (their) time of death. **Awful anxiety, anguish, great restlessness** with the **suddenness and violence** of the illness.

Marked congestion of the head and flushes of heat. Often needed in the first stage of high grade inflammations, fevers and congestions with great anxiety, heat and restlessness; tosses about, throws off the covers.

The senses are **oversensitive and burning pains** are characteristic but there may also be stinging, stabbing, tearing, cutting pains with numbness, tingling and crawling. **Intense pains**, neuralgic pains, cannot bear to be touched, in agony; worse (<) night and especially in the evening.

There is great **dryness and with it great thirst for cold water**. Characteristically the skin is dry and hot with no sweat. Worse (<) in a warm room and warm covers, better (>) uncovering; kicks off the covers.

Violent headaches which may be from exposure to a dry cold wind that has stopped a nasal catarrh from flowing.

Photophobia in fever with small contracted pupils.

Aconite is **bright red** in its inflammations, congested face, etc. though may turn pale on rising up. It is not dusky or mottled and it has no results of inflammation such as no suppuration, no thick green or yellow purulent discharges and no continued fever; *Aconite* is over quickly, in a night.

Everything may taste bitter, except water; They may crave bitter things in a fever. Burning, smarting and dryness of the throat with great redness and sometimes swelling.

Violent, sudden nausea and vomiting.

May go to sleep. The larynx becomes dry and they wake with spasms in the throat thinking they will choke. Croupy, choking, violent, dry cough with hoarse barking coming on in the night after being chilled in the day; intense febrile excitement. Suffocating cough. **Croup arising after exposure to cold, dry air**. Dry mucus membranes. A short dry cough, may be a little watery mucus, possibly blood streaked.

Other remedies will be needed if *Aconite* does not suffice and the condition lingers or continues on for more than a day or so. *Sulphur, Arnica, Belladonna, Bryonia, Ipecacuanha* follow it well.

Allium cepa

- Complaints often from cold, damp, penetrating winds

Complaints often from cold, damp, penetrating winds and it is **principally of use in colds and coughs**.

Copious watering of the eyes which is bland, watery nasal discharge which is acrid and excoriates the skin of the nose and upper lip are the strong characteristics of this remedy. All phases of the cold are worse

Allium cepa (continued)

- Principally of use in colds and coughs
- Copious watering of the eyes which is bland
- Watery nasal discharge which is acrid and excoriates the skin
- Worse (<) warmth, evenings

(<) **warmth** except the tickling in the larynx which can be worse (<) drawing in cold air.

(<) **Evenings** too. Coryza worse (<) indoors, better (>) open air.

Rawness of the mucous membranes. Tearing, painful larynx with each cough. Nose drips and burns with a sore upper lip and wings of the nose, red and raw. **Sneezing** comes early and with increasing frequency. Watery nasal discharge and obstruction goes from left to right nostril.

Much **congestion**; full, congestive headache often; fullness in the nose, may be throbbing and burning and sometimes nosebleeds.

Dull frontal headache, occipital headache; pain in the jaws go to the head. Severe headache sometimes and the eyes cannot stand the light. Tearing bursting and throbbing headaches. Headaches worse (<) in a warm room, better (>) in the open air like coryza.

Cough with tearing pains in the larynx, worse (<) drawing in cold air but also can be worse (<) in warm air or a warm room: worse (<) in the evening.

Spasmodic cough resembling croups or whooping cough; hoarse, harsh, ringing, spasmodic cough excited by constant tickling in the larynx. Cough that produces a raw, splitting sensation in the larynx that is so acute and severe that they make every effort not to cough.

Cold may also go down onto the chest with lots of secretions, coughing and rattling of mucus.

Antimonium tartaricum

- Chest complaints and gastric bowel disorders
- Face pale and sickly
- Feeble state, weakness, great drowsiness often
- Accumulation of mucus in the air passages
- Rattling breathing with the inability to raise phlegm
- Stomach troubles from sour food or drink
- Intense nausea
- Worse (<) lying down, warmth

This remedy is most often needed in chest complaints and gastric or bowel disorders. The face may be **pale and sickly** with dark rings round the eyes and may be covered in cold sweat. A state of relaxation and weakness with little fever, a lack of reactive power, a **feeble state, weakness, great drowsiness often.**

Every spell of cold, wet weather brings on coarse rattlings in the chest, a great **accumulation of mucus in the air passages**, or constant colds one after another. It lacks the vitality to throw these conditions off; it does not have the expulsive power of Ipecacuanha and the chest steadily fills up with mucus; **rattling breathing with the inability to raise phlegm**. May be sinking rapidly into this unreactive state; suffocating on white mucus; lacks the power to clear it but would be better (>) if they could.

They **must sit up** in bed, breathing is worse (<) **lying down**. They must be fanned sometimes but only slowly. They are worse (<) **warmth or too much clothing**, it makes them feel they are suffocating.

Mucous membranes covered in a thick white mucous exudate.

This weak, depleted state **does not come on early in an illness**. It comes with prostration, after several days and is most often found in patients of poor vitality, rather broken down weak constitutions who are subject to catarrhal illnesses; most often needed in the elderly and in young infants.

This person does not want to be meddled or interfered with in this state; everything is a burden and they do not want to be disturbed. The sick child does not want to be touched or sometimes even looked at. They want to be let alone. Pitiful, whining and moaning in the infant. Very irritable when disturbed. Occasionally may cling and want to be carried and may show their irritation in some other ways.

They may loathe food; even water is vomited.

Thirstless and usually is irritated if it is offered; the child only grunts. Sometimes there is a desire for cold things, acids or acid fruits which cause vomiting. **Stomach**

troubles from sour food or drink is another situation which may call for this remedy. Aversion to milk which is vomited. Vomiting, **intense nausea, prostration with coldness, cold sweat and drowsiness, sleepiness**. Vomiting ameliorates (>) the nausea unlike *Ipecacuanha*.

Apis mellifica

- Complaints come on quite rapidly
- Worse (<) heat or warm room
- Better (>) cold
- Pains sting and burn
- Marked rapid swelling
- Thirstlessness
- Face flushed, red
- Tightness throughout the abdomen, fear that something will burst
- Scanty urine
- Rashes feel rough
- Skin sensitive to touch

This remedy may be needed after a fright, rage, vexation, jealousy or hearing bad news. It may follow the disappearance or non-appearance of a rash, for instance if the rash of measles fails to develop fully or begins and then disappears.

Complaints come on quite rapidly in *Apis* like in *Belladonna*.

Worse (<) **heat or warm room** is very marked, this affects both the local conditions, like pains and inflammations, and also the patient himself; better (>) **cold in any form**, air, applications etc.

Complaints may start on the right and go to the left. **Pains characteristically sting and burn** and are better (>) **cold**; many other types of pain can occur though.

Swelling is also marked; rapid swelling, may come and go rapidly. Mucous membranes swollen as if filled with water even. Oedematous eyes, eylids, face or limbs.

Thirstlessness is also usual.

In delirium they may go into a stupor and even unconsciousness with twitchings sometimes, of one side; head rolling; pupils maybe contracted or dilated; eyes red; **face flushed, red**. Lying as if benumbed. May become deathly pale if the room is over-

heated; kick off the bed covers if they are able to.

Skin may be alternately hot and dry or perspiring.

A high pitched shriek or cry in a tossing or stuporose child.

Many eye complaints with burning tears, swelling and redness. Discharges sting and burn worse (<) heat and better (>) cold.

Suffocates from the radiated heat of a fire in a chill or fever.

Nausea of vomiting or retching with great anxiety.

Tightness throughout the abdomen making it impossible to cough or strain for **fear that something will burst** or will tear loose. They are likely to bend forward and flex the limbs in order to gain relief from the tightness. Very sore to touch.

Often there is **scanty urine**. There may be much urging to urinate, smarting, stinging, burning along the urinary tract.

Often needed in conditions where the skin is affected. **Rashes** feel thick, often **rough**; skin that is **sensitive to touch**, tender. Urticaria. Also may be worse (<) after sleep; touch.

Arnica

- Great bodily soreness as if bruised
- Greatly prostrated, weak and weary
- Averse to being talked to or even approached
- Hot and red head and face, cold extremities

The **great bodily soreness as if bruised** marks out *Arnica* (like *Baptisia*, *Phytolacca*, *Rhus tox.* and *Ruta*). The patient lies still, just turning a little from time to time. Why? Because of this soreness which make the bed feel too hard; it is no wonder that *Arnica* is the prime remedy for bruises and the results of trauma.

In fevers they may be **greatly prostrated, weak and weary**, stuporous, unconscious but can be aroused and will correctly answer your questions but will lapse back into this prostrate state. They may say they are not sick when clearly they are; this is because of the mental state. They want to be left alone; fear being touched because of the bodily soreness. **Averse to being talked to or even approached**; morose; irritable; sad; fearful; stupid; horror of instant death; nightmares, night horrors.

Hot and red head and face, cold extremities and body. Great thirst during the chill.

They have easy bleeding and bruising too; catarrhal complaints may be with inflamed mucous membranes which bleed easily.

In scarlet fever this state may come up when dusky, mottled and covered in red spots but the eruption does not come out (like *Antimonium tartaricum*).

Joints may be swollen and sore.

Offensiveness of eructations, taste, flatus and stool – smells like rotten eggs (*Baptisia* is even worse).

Sore as if bruised with a sore throat, consider *Phytolacca* which also has a hot red face and cold limbs and body.

Stupor with involuntary discharge of faeces and urine.

Many small boils, one after another, painful and sore.

Arsenicum album

- Anxiety
- Restlessness
- Weakness out of proportion to the illness
- Thirst for ice cold water, little and often, just sips
- Burning pains better (>) for heat
- Chilly
- Worse (<) for cold
- Worse (<) before and just after midnight
- Vomits everything
- Burns up and down
- Diarrhoea with exhaustion and restlessness

Anxiety, restlessness, weakness out of proportion to the illness, burning pains better (>) heat, foul odours, chilly, worse (<) before and just after midnight – these are characteristic of this remedy.

Worse (<) cold air or applications; usually chilly and better (>) warm wraps except for head complaints which are congestive and better (>) cool, fresh air. Often the skin is pale, cold and clammy.

Worse (<) movement, prostrated.

Anxiety is commonly intermingled with fear and takes the form of **restlessness**; it is a mental anxiety and uneasiness that makes the patient toss and turn, get up and walk about, move from place to place, one position to another but they become so weak that eventually, in very serious diseases, he

is prostrate even to having a deathly aspect. Commonly, he is too weak to move about as he would like to but if strong enough, he cannot keep still.

Thirst for ice cold water, little and often, just sips is another characteristic. They must drink because they are so dry yet cold water disagrees with their stomach so they only take it in sips. In stomach complaints he prefers warm things. In fevers there may be thirst for hot drinks during the chill, for sips during the heat and a copious thirst during the sweat. The sweat usually ameliorates (>) the condition (like *Natrum mur*).

Characteristically one finds chills with a sensation of ice water running in the blood vessels, this leads to an intensely hot fever with a sensation of boiling in the blood vessels, then comes the sweat and prostration with marked **chilliness**. Chilliness may alternate with flashes of heat too (like *Mercurius*).

Burning pains better (>) for heat is very characteristic of this remedy as is the weakness out of proportion to the illness.

Congestive, pulsating, burning in the head which is better (>) cold. All other burning pains elsewhere are better (>) heat, for example in the throat, stomach, lungs, bladder, eyes etc.

Discharges are acrid and cause burning better (>) heat.

A dry hacking cough and later a large quantity of thin watery or frothy mucus is expectorated. Burning in the chest. Difficulty with breathing, wheezy; must sit up to breath and is much worse (<) for any exertion.

Vomits everything with the prostration and anxiety, dry mouth, burning pains better (>) heat, better (>) warm water or milk **burns up and down**. Gastritis. A very sensitive stomach better (>) heat. Diarrhoea and vomiting simultaneously, worse (<) after eating or drinking. **Diarrhoea with exhaustion and restlessness**, better (>) heat; foul smell. Rectum and anus burn and become raw and excoriated.

Mentally may be oversensitive, fussy and fastidious. Sensitive to smell and touch.

Chilly, always taking colds which cause catarrh and sneezing; from every change in the weather. Catarrhs travel down to the larynx and hoarseness, to the trachea with burning worse (<) for coughing and to the chest with constriction and a cough.

Belladonna

- Complaints come on suddenly and with great violence
- Violent heat
- Redness – bright, shiny red skin
- Intense burning in the inflamed parts
- Swelling
- Very sensitive to pains which come and go suddenly
- Congestion with throbbing all over
- Hot head and cold extremities
- Great dryness of mucus membranes

Like *Aconite* it is suited to plethoric, vigorous, healthy constitutions, robust children and babies when the complaints come on **suddenly and with great violence**, then subsides just as suddenly; a short, sharp course – **Not** to be used in prolonged, continuous or recurrent states or in complaints which come on gradually.

Great liability to take cold; sensitive to a draught especially on the head like *Hepar sulph.* and *Silica*.

Violent heat, so intense that it lingers on the hand after touching the patient's skin. All sorts of inflammations and fevers.

Redness – bright, shiny red skin especially of face, mucous membranes etc. Later it may become a little dusky and mottled.

Burning – intense burning in the inflamed parts. The throat burns like coals of fire; the skin burns in scarlet fever and inflammations; gastritis burns.

Swelling – inflamed parts swell rapidly, are very sensitive to touch with the sensation as if they would burst, with pressing, stinging, burning pains.

Very sensitive to pains, which **come and go suddenly**. Much suffering; **worse (<) motion, jar**, cold, touch, pressure, light. They want to be warmly wrapped unlike Apis.

Congestion with throbbing all over and burning; blood vessels throb and pulsate as do local inflammations; hammering pains in the head if they move. The more congestion there is the more excitability. In fever they become **delirious**, see horrible faces, animals, etc.; a wild state even, which is sometimes better (>) eating some light food. Vertigo is common.

Congestive headache worse (<) stooping, lying down; wants to wrap up the head. Marked congestion predominates in head symptoms; a sense of fullness.

Belladonna (continued)

- Dry skin but often sweats on covered parts
- Twitching and jerking, starts and jumps in fevers
- Worse (<) motion
- Worse (<) at 3pm and at night

Hot head and cold extremities; rush of blood to the head. Eyes red and bloodshot.

Burning dryness and sense of constriction in the throat. **Great dryness of mucous membranes** with copious thirst or may be thirstless; often craves lemons or lemonade in fevers. **Dry skin but often sweats on covered parts.**

Tongue may have red edges and white central coating. Offensive, putrid taste.

Twitching and jerking, starts and jumps – more common in fevers, even to convulsions. Restless sleep, full of dreams of violence, nightmares, moaning and groaning.

Dryness produces tickling, leading to a dry, barking cough; violent cough and may produce a little blood stained mucus. Once mucus is raised there is relief for a while and then it repeats. Chest very sore and tight, children may cry before they cough. Tickling and burning in the larynx with violent paroxysms of coughing. Headache as if head would burst with the cough.

Tendency to right sided complaints and cannot lie on the painful side unlike *Bryonia*.

Most complaints are better (>) keeping still; frequently **worse (<) at 3 pm and at night.**

Bryonia

- Complaints come on slowly, are continuous or remittent
- Much worse (<) motion
- Worse (<) heat and stuffy rooms
- Better (>) pressure
- Extreme irritability
- A sluggish state of mind
- Headache accompanies almost all other illnesses
- Stitching pains and lies on the painful side
- Chest painful and they hold it when coughing
- Dryness of mucous membranes
- Great thirst for large quantities of cold water

Complaints begin a day or more after taking cold, especially if overheated or if the sweat is suppressed by cold air or water, or from exposure to dry cold winds. They may also follow some mortification or hurt feelings.

Complaints often commence in the morning and may follow several days of preparation – feeling languid, tired, stupid in the head – and may increase gradually into violence. **Complaints come on slowly, are continuous or remittent**. Often suited to plethoric, slow people subject to catarrhal congestions.

Much worse (<) motion is always present. They desire to keep perfectly still; the more and the longer they move the more they suffer.

Better (>) **Pressure**, it holds the parts still.

Extreme irritability; does not want to talk or be disturbed and may later be stupefied, a state of stupor bordering on unconsciousness even. **A sluggish state of mind**, not excitable; when roused from stupor they may be confused, want to go home etc., a low type of delirium, **not** the flashing wild excitement of *Belladonna*. Delirium may start at 9 pm and last all night like the fever. Chill at 9 pm too.

9 pm is a common time of aggravation for *Bryonia* complaints.

They may be indecisive and not know what they want. Sometimes their anxiety and an uneasy feeling compel them to move like *Arsenicum* and, even though it makes the pains worse (<), they cannot keep still; or the pains can be so violent that they also have to move but it still makes the pains worse (<).

Worse (<) heat, better (>) cold. In themselves and their congestive complaints they are worse (<) heat and better (>) cold (like *Apis*, *Pulsatilla* etc.) Some rheumatic complaints are better (>) heat though.

Headache may be on its own or **the forerunner of other complaints; it accompanies almost all other illnesses.** There may be mental dullness and confusion with a bursting headache; usually better (>) tight pressure. Headache with nausea, with faintness. Splitting, violent, congestive headache, a pressure pain; headache as if the skull would split. Worse (<) motion, even the winking of an eye; exertion is impossble, they keep perfectly quiet and still, in the dark too because worse (<) by light. Worse (<) **heat and stuffy rooms**, stooping, sitting up after lying down, coughing. Often looks rather besotted with a congested mottled and purple face; a bloated face but not oedema.

Stitching pains (like *Kali carb.*) **and lies on the painful side** (unlike *Belladonna* or *Kali carb.*); lies still and is better (>) pressure. They hold their heads tight when coughing because of the splitting headache.

Many complaints start in the nose with sneezing, coryza with red eyes and headache. It may progress to the throat, larynx and down onto the chest. Burning and tickling of the larynx, hoarseness and congestion of the chest. They feel sore, lame and bruised all over (*Arnica* more so). The **chest** may be **painful and they hold it when coughing** and lie on the painful side to keep it still and put pressure on it. A chill with much pain in the chest, a short, hard, racking, dry cough with scanty or rusty coloured sputum. They take short rapid breaths because of the pain on deeper inspiration; pleurisy. Affinity for the right side with pain and pneumonia. A violent cough racks the body sometimes with a headache and copious mucus. Cough worse (<) after eating, movement, going from cold to warm air.

Dryness of mucous membranes, from lips to anus. Lips very dry, children tend to pick them; mouth dry.

Great thirst for large quantities of cold water at long intervals.

Toothache better (>) cold and pressure. There may be loss of or altered taste with a dry brown tongue and even, rarely, thirstlessness. Dry sore throat with the thirst but cold drinks may bring on the cough and pains. In stomach complaints warm drinks ameliorate (>).

Thickly coated white tongue. Sore throats with aphthous ulceration.

They may crave what their stomach is averse to; indecisive. Sitting up may cause nausea and faintness. Disordered digestion with the sensation of a stone or weight in the stomach (like *Nux vomica*, *Pulsatilla* etc). Bitter taste in the mouth (like *Pulsatilla*, *Nux vomica* is sour). Nausea and vomiting worse (<) motion. Complaints follow errors in the diet especially at the beginning of a warm spell after cold weather. Constipation with dry, hard stools is most characteristic but also may get diarrhoea worse (<) morning, movement and from overeating.

All complaints are usually better (>) sweat. Generally worse (<) after eating, at 9 pm. Pains, except in the abdomen are better (>) pressure.

Calcarea carbonica

- Complaints may follow exposure to cold water
- Full of congestions
- A chilly patient; sensitive to cold air
- Coldness with sweats.
- Sweats in spots

Complaints may follow exposure to cold water.

Full of **congestions**. Cold feet and hot head.

A chilly patient; sensitive to cold air, raw winds, a draught, a storm. **Takes cold so easily. Coldness** of parts especially lower legs and feet. Worse (<) cold air, ascending or exertion.

Coldness with sweats. Sweats in spots, in various places; head, forehead, back of neck, front of chest, feet. If they get into a sweat and stop still too long the sweat will stop suddenly and they get a chill or a headache.

Relaxed tissues and blood vessels – varicose veins, piles etc. with burning in varicose veins.

Calcarea carbonica (continued)

- Relaxed tissues and blood vessels
- Weakness
- Glands, especially lymph nodes, hard, inflamed and sore
- Sourness
- Sweats about the head on the least exertion
- Hot head during congestions

Weakness, worse (<) exertion, out of breath. Fever or headache from exertion.

Glands, especially lymph nodes, become **hard, inflamed and sore**. Abscesses in deep tissues.

Sourness; sour vomiting, diarrhoea, smell of the body, breath etc. Tendency to looseness of the bowels worse (<) afternoon.

Tired and exhausted mentally and physically; break down in a sweat and become excited and irritable. Complaints lasting for days or weeks from excitement of the emotions, worry or vexation. Inability to apply themselves.

Sweats about the head on the least exertion, covered with cold sweat. Sweats on forehead and every draught of air chills and brings on a headache. Feet sweat, cold and damp. Neck sweats at night.

Hot head during congestions.

Headaches are stupefying, benumbing and bring on confusion of mind. Headache from suppressed coryza. Pulsating headache if severe.

The more marked the congestion of the internal parts the colder the surface becomes.

Cold, icy, sweaty hands with chest, stomach and bowel complaints. Fever with cold sweat on the scalp. Burning in vertex of head with coldness in the forehead. Sweaty head at night which wets the pillow.

Thick yellow discharge from ears or nose after cold weather.

Sore throats in those that take cold frequently, one straight after another; chronic sore throats with constant dry, choking feeling with pain on swallowing. Painless hoarseness, worse (<) morning.

Colds all settle on the chest, so tired; expectoration of thick, yellow mucus, may be sour, offensive. Cough is better (>) cold, wet, wind.

Weak, sensitive back; slides down in the bed.

Rheumatic joints, stiffness on rising from a seat.

Sleep disturbed by ideas, horrible visions on closing the eyes; grinds teeth, chews and swallows. Cold feet in bed and when they warm up they burn and need cooling.

Causticum

- The Causticum cough
- Dry, raw, hoarse even to complete loss of voice
- Tracheal irritation

This gives the picture of the Causticum cough:

Rawness and tickling in the throat with a dry cough. Burning in the throat not better (>) swallowing. **Dry, raw, hoarse** even to complete loss of voice; **hoarseness worse (<) mornings**.

Hard, dry cough racks the whole chest. Tracheal irritation – a raw streak down the centre of the upper chest.

Chest seems to be full of mucus, if only they could cough a little deeper they feel they would be able to shift it and get it up. Struggle and cough until exhausted or until they find that a little cold drink will relieve. Cough worse (<) expiration.

Leak of urine may occur with each cough. Soreness in the chest with the cough.

Inability to expectorate and is obliged to swallow any sputum that is raised; it may taste greasy.

Dry cough with pain in the hip, involuntary urination.

Chamomilla

- Great sensitivity especially to pain
- Great irritability and oversensitiveness
- Angry, snarling crying; piteous moaning
- Teething

Great sensitivity especially to pain, also to impressions, surroundings and persons.

Great irritability and oversensitiveness. Cross, ugly, spiteful and snappish.

This state may arise from anger, a temper, being contradicted, feeling mortified or from physical pain itself.

Angry, snarling crying; piteous moaning. These states are often found in the child and it is this emotional picture that will usually indicate the remedy. They may be driven to a frenzy by the pains, with a total loss of consideration for others; they may be quarrelsome, disputative and uncivil. Children are often snappish and cannot be touched; they want to do as they please yet do not know what pleases them! A spunky, peevish state that can occur with inflammation anywhere. They may whine and cry; sputter about everything; not know what they want and are never satisfied, capriciously rejecting the things they have just asked for and such a **temper**.

Sometimes better (>) for passive motion; they want to be carried the whole time but even then they may not be quietened for long and will demand to be carried by someone else.

With earache children may screech out, cannot keep still with the pain and may be violently excited by it. Earache may be very sensitive to the cold. **Very sensitive to pain** which makes them mad, cannot bear the pain, sweats with the pains. Sometimes there is numbness with the pains.

Thirsty for cold water usually. High fever with sweating especially on the head, one cheek red and one pale.

Very useful in **teething** which is this oversensitive, capricious state where nothing pleases and the teething is worse (<) heat and night, better (>) cold applications. Teething with green, foul diarrhoea smelling of rotten eggs and there may be colicky pain and bloating.

Most complaints come on in the evening or night and subside by midnight usually. May be worse (<) 9 am. Often worse (<) heat but not better (>) cold in general, (unlike *Pulsatilla* and *Apis*). In fact cold may bring on most troubles.

Drosera

- A remedy for coughs that are spasmodic
- A dry cough with tickling
- Worse (<) lying down and after midnight

A remedy for coughs that are spasmodic, that is with spasm and constrictions; painful and often exhausting. A dry cough with tickling.

Worse (>) lying down and after midnight, drinking and eating.

The pains in the chest are better (>) pressure.

A tickling cough coming every few hours with increasing intensity. It may lead to vomiting or haemorrhage. Tickling or crawling in the larynx provokes cough and wakes them.

Constriction felt in the throat, larynx or chest with the spasmodic cough, can hardly get any breath; suffocation with the spasms in the chest and larynx and the constant violent paroxysms of coughing, worse (<) lying down. Constriction preventing swallowing. Clutching, cramping, burning felt in the larynx.

Deep sounding hoarse cough; tenacious mucus or dry.

Coughing spasms every 2–3 hours worse (<) lying down at night until 3 am.

Stitching pains in the chest worse (<)

coughing and better (>) pressure, they hold the chest like *Bryonia*. Pain in top of abdomen better (>) holding it while coughing.

Chill and fever worse (<) after midnight; cold copious sweat; hot head and cold extremities; no thirst.

They may have shivering at rest better (>) motion.

They feel generally better (>) in the open air.

Dulcamara

- Strong affinity for catarrhal states of mucus membrane
- Every change of the weather, especially from warm to cold
- From perspiration that is checked
- From taking cold
- Norse (<) cold wet weather

This remedy has a strong affinity for **catarrhal states** of mucous membranes.

It is often caused by **every change of the weather, especially from warm to cold; from perspiration that is checked** especially if hot; **from taking cold; from cold wet weather.**

They are **worse (<) cold, damp weather**, worse (<) in the Autumn, in the evening and night, at rest. They are better (>) for dry even weather, for motion, for rising from a seat, for warmth.

In diarrhoea which comes on when there are hot days and cold nights and the nature of the stools keeps changing (like *Pulsatilla*). Infant diarrhoea may be like this. There are yellow or yellowy green, slimy and undigested stools. Frequently there is a mass of slimy substance. **Diarrhoeas** that come on **after taking cold.**

Back and neck pains and stiffness from cold and damp.

Fevers may come on from going into cold air whilst hot; with trembling, aching bones and muscles; a dazed state, they cannot remember things.

Sore catarrhal eyes from taking cold.

There is a tendency for mucous membranes to ulcerate and the ulcers to spread.

Sore throat every time they breathe cold air when overheated, especially if it is cold damp air.

Urge to urinate may come if the patient becomes chilled.

There may be dry, teasing winter coughs; dry, rough and hoarse or a loose cough with copious mucus worse (<) lying, in a warm room, better (>) in the open air.

Cold sores may appear on the lips or genitalia.

Eupatorium perfoliatum

- Aching in bones as if they would break

Aching in bones as if they would break is the main feature of this remedy that accompanies all of its complaints. It is otherwise very similar to *Bryonia*.

Winter colds with much sneezing, coryza and headache as if it would burst which is **worse (<)** motion, in a person who is chilly and wants to be warmly wrapped and has

Eupatorium perfoliatum (continued)

- Winter colds with much sneezing, coryza and headache as if it would burst
- Chill at 7–9 am intense aching in bones before the chill
- Worse (<) motion

much aching in the bones. There can be fever, thirst and generally worse (<) for motion. After a few days it may go onto their chest or settle in the liver causing a bilious fever and even jaundice.

An attack may begin with the sensation as if their back were breaking, great shivering all over, a congestive headache and flushed face. A high fever; bilious vomiting and those aching bones. There may be stomach pains after eating. The patient wants to keep still but the pains can be so severe that they must move so sometimes they can appear to be restless.

In the chest they may have a dry racking, teasing, hacking cough and so sore and worse (<) motion; it is similar to *Bryonia* and *Phosphorus*. Hoarseness in the morning with a sore aching chest.

They are very sensitive to cold air, as much as in *Nux vomica* which also has the aching bones and wants to be covered and in a hot room. *Nux vomica* has dreadful irritability of temper whereas *Eupatorium* tends towards overwhelming sadness.

Chill at 7–9 am. Intense aching in bones before the chill. There is often a thirst but during the chill cold water often makes this worse (<). Vomiting often comes at the close of a chill; vomiting of bile between the chill and the heat. They burn all over with the heat and feel hotter than their temperature would justify. There is usually little sweat. A violent headache may be present during the chill and it can be worse (<) sweat. Fever every third day too.

Euphrasia

- Marked affinity for the eyes
- In fevers the chills predominate
- A catarrhal remedy; catarrhal headaches
- Profuse, watery, excoriating discharge from the eyes with a bland, fluent discharge from the nose
- Worse (<) daytime
- Better (>) lying down
- No cough at night

Marked affinity for the eyes.

A chilly person who cannot get warm. In fevers the **chills predominate** with the fever mostly in the day, red faced with cold hands. Often the perspiration is confined to the upper part of the body.

A catarrhal remedy; catarrhal headaches; often has a headache with eye complaints or coryza; a bursting, bruised headache with dazzling from bright lights; headache in the evening.

Catarrh may be with or without fever.

A tendency to accumulate sticky mucus on the cornea removed by blinking.

Profuse, watery, excoriating discharge from the eyes with a bland, fluent discharge from the nose is a very strong symptom for this remedy.

Dry, burning, biting, pressure in the eyes, as if by dust with itching. Swollen mucous

membranes, red and enlarged blood vessels; inflammation of all the tissues of the eye. Contracted pupils. There may be a purulent discharge too. Many tears in cold air and windy weather. The lids may be very sensitive and swollen; the margins itch and burn. Blepharitis. A fine rash about the eyes. Pain in the eyes is worse (<) open air and light. Lots of tears.

Sneezing and fluent, bland coryza; the mucous membranes of the nose may be swollen and after a day or two the coryza may extend to the larynx with a hard cough.

Coryza is worse (<) lying down at night and worse (<) in the open air and windy weather.

Cough is **worse (<) daytime and is better (>) lying down**. It sometimes comes on in the open air. There may be hoarseness in the morning; irritation in the larynx compelling them to cough, followed by pressure beneath the sternum. Abundant secretions in the larynx causing a loose cough with rattling in the chest; copious expectoration with or after the coryza. Difficulty breathing may be better (>) lying down at night and worse (<) in the morning when there may be copious and usually easy expectoration. **No cough at night, like in *Bryonia*.** Usually loose but sometimes can be a dry cough.

Ferrum phosphoricum

- Complaints come on often from overexertion.
- The early stages of many illnesses
- Great weakness and the desire to lie down
- Haemorrhagic complaints
- Nosebleeds
- Worse (<) open air
- Better (>) gentle motion

The onset is not quite as rapid or violent as *Belladonna* or *Aconite* but it is not quite as torpid and slow as *Gelsemium*. Complaints come on often from overexertion.

Great weakness and the desire to lie down is a strong feature as are **haemorrhagic complaints**; problems involving some sort of bleeding. There may be fainting spells but the patient is more alert than in *Belladonna*. There are congestions and a vascular fullness, pulsations and surgings of blood. Flushes of the face and a flushed face – a false kind of plethora that is often confined to well described circular patches on the cheeks. Their appearance may not be one of illness because of these pink cheeks.

There may be nervousness at night, trembling limbs, though not as anxious as *Aconite*. Sometimes they are loquacious and mirthful when ill. Often the mind is confused when trying to think, difficulty concentrating and they can become forgetful, dull and indifferent as they tire, better (>) for cold washing of the face.

They are sensitive to the open air and worse (<) from it; always taking cold.

Soreness throughout the body is worse (<) jar and walking. Many complaints are worse (<) from lying in bed and from rest and are better (>) slowly moving about but the great lassitude compels them to lie down. Restless at night with the fever, for ever tossing about.

There may be numbness of affected parts, stitching, tearing pains and may be oversensitive to pain.

Ear infections with a purulent discharge, itching and noises in the ears; eustachian catarrh.

Coryza may be acrid and purulent or a bloody discharge. **Nosebleeds** may come with the coryza, with fear or a headache when the head is congested, hot and full.

Dry lips with a flushed face. Dry cough which is worse (<) for cold, eating and deep breathing, with a mucous coryza or dryness. Sore chest or stitching pain with the cough or deep breathing. Mucus of all sorts.

Backache, a stiff neck, wry neck.

Chills in the afternoon and at night, a shaking chill. Fever has a dry heat with thirst, flushes of heat and perspiration.

Cold extremities or heat all over.

They may desire sour things but are worse (<) for them.

Worse (<) open air; physical exertion, after eating; cold drinks; sour food; standing.

They are better (>) **for gentle motion** like *Pulsatilla*.

Gelsemium

- Complaints may follow fear, shock, embarrassment or fright
- Insidious onset
- Slow, congestive complaints and headache
- Congestion of the head is most marked
- A feeling of great weight and tiredness
- Dazed and talk as if delirious, incoherent, stupid, forgetful
- Face flushed, dusky
- Mottled skin
- Cold extremities with hot head and back
- Chills run up and down back
- Little thirst
- Disturbed sensations

The complaints of *Gelsemium* may follow fear, shock, embarrassment or fright.

There is an **insidious onset** of complaints, several days after exposure or shock etc. Colds and fevers are of a low grade, **not violent. Slow, congestive complaints and headaches. Congestion of the head is most marked**. It is suited to the warmer climates and milder winters.

A feeling of great weight and tiredness runs all through the remedy; so **weary and heavy** that they must lie down and lie still. Trembling if they attempt to move. Children may have a fear of falling, in fevers, and hold on tight. They are in a state of nervous excitement when awake though they lie thinking of nothing in particular because their minds will not work in an orderly way. They may be **dazed and talk as if delirious, incoherent, stupid, forgetful**; worse (<) for mental exertions and is averse to speaking or even having company present; too tired to communicate and not wanting to make the effort.

Congestive headaches with most violent pain in the occiput, sometimes hammering, pulsating pain. So violent sometimes that they cannot stand up but lie perfectly exhausted. Often better (>) by lying still, bolstered up by pillows. Better (>) pressure and alcohol, it stimulates them; worse (<) mental exertion, smoking, lying with the head low, heat of the sun. **Face flushed, dusky**, mind dazed, eyes glassy, pupils often dilated, cold extremities, **mottled skin**, scanty urine, cramps in fingers, toes and back.

Dizziness with blurred or double vision.

Cold extremities with hot head and back; face purple during congestion, high fever. **Great coldness and chills run up and down the back**; pains can go up the back too. Chattering teeth and shaking even without a sense of coldness. High fever in the afternoons may progress to a continued fever with **little thirst** and marked head complaints, a dazed mind etc. They are as still as in *Bryonia* but it is because they are so tired and weary, not from the pain and their head is more congested than in *Bryonia*. Profuse, exhaustive sweats, too weak to move.

Coryza with sneezing and a watery discharge, cold extremities. It goes down to the throat with redness and swelling, enlarged tonsils, hot head, congested face, **heavy limbs**, a gradual onset.

There may be tearing pains in nerves, sciatica, numbness, **disturbed sensations**.

Disturbance of vision before attacks; double, dim, misty vision or nystagmus.

Palpitations with fever. A sense of weakness or goneness in the heart region that extends to the stomach creating a sensation of hunger. The heart's pulse is feeble, soft and irregular, (unlike *Aconite*, *Belladonna* etc.)

Paralytic states of sphincters – involuntary stool and urination. Weakness of extremities or just awkward and clumsy. **Ptosis**.

Diarrhoea from sudden excitement or emotion, bad news, fright, anticipation of some ordeal.

In summary – great heaviness and weakness of the limbs, congested head, face flushed, mottled, dusky red or purple, cold extremities, dazed and delirious, stuporose, with disturbances of sensations and paralysed sphincters coming on slowly.

Hepar sulphuris

- Chilly, irritable and hypersensitive.
- From exposure to dry cold winds
- The least uncovering of a hand or foot causes chilliness
- Oversensitive to impressions, touch, surroundings, cold and pain
- Quarrelsome, nothing pleases, everything disturbs
- Catarrhal states
- Sweating all night without relief
- Worse (<) cold
- Better (>) heat and wet weather

Chilly, irritable and hypersensitive.

From exposure to dry cold winds or after the premature disappearance of a rash.

All the complaints are worse (<) **cold**. They want the room warm and to be well covered. **The least uncovering of a hand or foot causes chilliness** or cough.

Oversensitive to impressions, touch, surroundings, cold and pain. Intense suffering even without apparently sufficient cause. Pains are severe, sharp and sticking; very sensitive inflammations and ulcerations. Splinter pains in the throat worse (<) from swallowing. They may even faint with the pains.

Delicate oversensitive people who become **extremely irritable**. Angry, abusive and impulsive. **Quarrelsome, nothing pleases, everything disturbs**. Desires a constant change of people, surroundings or things.

Tendency to suppuration with this irritability – glands, ulcers, boils, injuries.

Catarrhal states; coryza with much sneezing and obstruction every time they go into a cold wind. Initially watery, later thick, yellow and offensive smelling often like decomposed cheese. **All discharges can smell of decomposed cheese, or may smell sour**.

Copious catarrhs of the throat and pharynx; **splinter pains**; extremely sensitive to touch; pain on swallowing.

Loss of voice and dry hoarse bark, especially in the mornings and the evenings, worse (<) cold and dry winds, worse (<) uncovering.

A great remedy in **croup** for sensitive children who have been exposed to cold air or **dry cold winds** and have come down with croup the following morning (see also *Aconite* and *Spongia* particularly); worse (<) morning and evening. It may follow *Aconite* if an attack returns the next morning. The more rattling there is in the chest the more it is like *Hepar*. There may be a loose cough in the day and a dry paroxysmal cough in the evening and night.

The catarrhal state may be lower down in the trachea which becomes extremely sore from much coughing for days and weeks, again is worse (<) morning and evening, a rattling, wheezing, barking cough in an oversensitive, chilly patient. They may cough and sweat; much sweating throughout the night which does not relieve.

Sweating all night without relief is found in many complaints. Sweats easily. *Hepar* may be needed after *Mercurius*.

Ear infections with a bloody, purulent, cheesy smelling discharge and sticking pains. Offensive thick eye discharges too.

They may hate fat and love vinegar, pickles and other sour things, spices, strong tasting foods. Sourness like in *Calcarea carbonica*.

Heat and wet weather, damp.

Worse (<) lying on the painful side, touch, pressure, motion, exertion, tight clothing.

Ipecacuanha

- Rapid onset over a few hours
- Nausea and vomiting runs right through this remedy

Rapid onset over a few hours.

Nausea and vomiting runs right through this remedy especially if the **vomiting does not relieve the nausea**. Often an acute complaint begins with **nausea and vomiting** with a **clean tongue**. The stomach and bowels feel relaxed as if hanging down.

Prostration comes in spells, unlike *Arsenicum* where it is continuous.

Complaints may come on from suppressed

Ipecacuanha (continued)

- Vomiting does not relieve the nausea
- Prostration comes in spells
- Bronchitis of children with coarse rattling, coughing, gagging and a sense of suffocation
- Desire fresh air very much

emotions or vexations. Nausea from eating rich foods, like in *Pulsatilla*, and after dietary indulgences.

Violent chills, face flushed bright red or bluish red.

Colds settle in the nose which may stuff up at night with much sneezing and blows out mucus and often blood; nosebleeds with every cold. Colds descend and produce hoarseness then rawness of the trachea, then to the chest with suffocation and a great accumulation of mucus but there is an expulsive power to the cough (unlike in *Antimonium tartaricum*).

Dry, teasing, hacking cough with a sense of suffocation. They choke and gag and get red in the face. Bloody sputum. Whooping cough may be like this or even asthma.

Bronchitis of children with **coarse rattling, coughing, gagging and a sense of suffocation**, weight and anxiety in the chest, after a rapid onset and they look dreadfully sick, drawn and pale; the condition has come on rapidly. Mucus in the chest and it will not come up, rattling and wheezing.

Wheeziness which is like this and is worse (<) damp weather, better (>) sitting up and for fresh air. Often they **desire fresh air very much**. Cough with inclination to vomit without nausea; usually intense nausea though.

Generally thirstless except in the fever which is prolonged and with nausea.

Headache as if bruised all through the bones of the head and down into the root of the tongue with nausea. Nausea may precede the headache.

Dysentery like diarrhoea with awful tenesmus; they may pass a little blood or green slime. **Constant nausea**; vomit bile; vomit everything taken in, with great prostration and great pallor. Copious diarrhoea often of green slime or mucus. Much crying and straining at stool in the infant. Colic with nausea and green stools; fermented, foamy stools.

Worse (<) damp, overeating.

Better (>) open air, rest.

Kali bichromicum

- Catarrhal remedy
- Copious, ropy, mucus discharges from mucous membranes anywhere
- Wandering pains and very severe pains in small spots
- Always suffering with or nasal Catarrh
- Better (>) warmth
- Worse (<) morning

This is a **catarrhal remedy**. There may be **copious, ropy, mucus discharges from mucous membranes anywhere**; great long string of mucus; jelly-like mucus.

The catarrhal symptoms may alternate with joint symptoms and rheumatic pains in the winter. In the summer, diarrhoea alternates with rheumatic complaints.

Wandering pains (like *Pulsatilla*) **and very severe pains in small spots**, such as can be covered by a thumb tip, are characteristic. Sharp, stitching pains too. Pains often appear and disappear rapidly (like *Belladonna*).

A chilly person, everywhere, especially in the back of the neck. Pains and cough are **better (>) warmth**.

Always suffering with a nasal catarrh; pressing pain in the root of the nose with a chronic catarrh and if exposed to the cold the discharge dries up and a headache begins, (like in *Kali carbonicum*), often starting with dim vision. The pains may be pulsating, shooting, burning, better (>) for warmth and pressure. One sided pains or even just in spots. Often retching and vomiting occur with the headache and sometimes vertigo; **worse (<) morning**, night, motion, stooping.

Kali bichromicum (continued)

Very red inflamed throat with swollen tonsils, swollen neck and even suppuration; with this the pain extends to the ears. There may be a dry burning sensation; a dry mouth, ropy mucus, mouth ulcers. The uvula can be oedematous. Intense pain in the root of the tongue on protrusion may be present or the sensation of a hair on the tongue. Yellow coating at the base of the tongue or a dry, smooth, glazed, cracked tongue.

Copious, thick, ropy mucus from the larynx; hoarseness, rough voice, dry cough. Cough worse (<) breathing, worse (<) damp cold weather and may be better (>) in a warm bed at night. Stitching pain with the cough. Much wheezing and tightness in the centre of the chest. There is a charactristic pain from the sternum to the back with the catarrh and the cough. A tickling, dry, hard cough; great soreness in the chest on coughing or deep breathing. Hard coughing on waking, better (>) lying down, warm bed, worse (<) cold air, undressing, deep breathing. Ropy, yellow or green mucus with rattling in the chest.

Digestion is suspended and their food lies like a load in the stomach; fullness and distress come on immediately after eating. Much foetid eructations. Averse to meat and they may desire beer which produces vomiting and diarrhoea.

Worse (<) 2–3 am, in the morning, for motion.

Ulcers of mucous membranes can be deep as if punched out.

Kali carbonicum

- Sensitive to every draught or air movement
- Stitching pains
- Pains that fly around
- Worse (<) 3–5 am
- Dry, hacking, barking cough in cold air
- Swelling between eyelids and eyebrows

These people are worse (<) wet weather and worse (<) cold weather. They tend to be sensitive to every change in the atmosphere; they cannot get the temperature exactly right. **Sensitive to every draught or air movement**.

Sensitive to cold, always shivering. Their nerves may be painful when cold and if the affected part is kept warm the pain goes to some other place that is uncovered.

Stitching pains, burning, tearing pains. **Pains that fly around**, wander from place to place.

Worse (<) 3–5 am.

Catarrhal, congestive headaches from cold air which clears the nose and brings on a headache (like *Kali bich.*). In a warm room the nose discharges and fills up which ameliorates the headache; a thick, fluent, yellow discharge.

There is a tendency for colds to locate in the chest.

Dry cough day and night with vomiting of food and some phlegm, worse (<) after eating and drinking, worse (<) evenings.

Chronic bronchitis. Dryness, a dry, hacking, barking cough in cold air, which is when they feel most uncomfortable; copious expectoration of mucus in the warm which produces a general amelioration. Expectoration may be very offensive, tenacious, lumpy, blood streaked or like thick, yellow or yellow/green pus, often with a pungent, cheesy taste. Mostly they have a dry hacking cough with morning expectoration, increasing to a most violent, gagging cough with vomiting and a sensation as if their head would burst or fly to pieces. The face begins to swell and the eyes to protrude with the cough and then comes **oedema** between the eyelids and the eyebrows, even to the extent of a little water bag forming.

Wheeziness worse (<) 3–5 am, better (>) leaning forward or by rocking, like *Arsenicum*; with rattling in the chest, rattling cough and stitches in the chest with respiration, like *Bryonia*, or between breaths. Sputum of small round lumps.

Pain in the lower right chest through to the back (like *Mercurius*) worse (<) lying on the painful side, (opposite to *Bryonia*).

Great flatulence, everything eaten turns to gas.

Lachesis

- Worse (<) on waking
- Sleep into an aggravation
- Worse (<) spring time or on going from cold to warm, becoming warm
- Better (>) onset of a discharge
- Surging waves of pain
- Face is congested, mottled, purplish and engorged
- Complaints on the left side or go from left to right
- Neck is very sensitive to touch

The modalities are likely to lead to this remedy:

Complaints are **worse (<) on waking**, they **sleep into an aggravation** (<).

Worse (<) light touch or pressure.

Worse (<) spring time or on going from cold to warm, becoming warm, they cannot breath in the heat.

Better (>) onset of a discharge eg. menses or a nasal catarrh.

Surging waves of pain and the face is **congested, mottled, purplish and engorged**. Puffed eyelids and face. Inflamed parts take on a bluish, purplish tint.

They hate constrictions about the neck or abdomen.

Complaints are characteristically on the **left side or go from left to right**.

Headache on waking, sleeps into it. Face very pale with the headache. Waves of pain worse (<) after moving. Bursting, pulsating headache, **pressure and burning on the vertex** and the senses are overwrought; worse (<) noise, cannot stand the touch of the clothes, especially about the neck. Dim vision and flickerings with the headache and a very pale face, maybe vertigo. Relief often comes with a discharge such as the menses or a nasal discharge etc.

Dyspnoea; they wake from sleep with a sense of suffocation, a sense of choking which can come on in the first sleep, a sense of strangulation when lying and especially when anything is around the neck; **neck is very sensitive to touch**. They wake with this sense of suffocation and must sit up and bend forward or else must rush to the open window; they feel they must take a deep breath.

The cough is dry, suffocating like *Spongia* and tickling. Little secretion and much sensitiveness, worse (<) pressure on larynx; larynx is painful to touch. Cough **worse (<) after sleep** like *Spongia*; coughs early in sleep at about 11 pm.

Throat problems are worse (<) empty swallowing or swallowing liquids, solids usually go down much easier. Throat pains go to the ears and are worse (<) for hot drinks, (unlike *Lycopodium*). Painful hawking of mucus. Starts on left and goes to right. Purplish hue to the inflammation. Throat and neck sensitive to the slightest touch.

Lycopodium

- Complaints are right sided, go from right to left or above downwards
- A chilly patient with pains better (>) warmth except the head complaints which are better (>) cold and worse (<) in a warm room
- Sore throats better for warm drinks
- Great flatulence and belching
- Often worse (<) 4–8 pm
- Full and distended after very few mouthfuls

Complaints are **right sided**, go from **right to left or above downwards.**

A chilly patient with pains **better (>) warmth except the head complaints which are better (>) cold and worse (<) in a warm room.**

Often worse (<) 4–8 pm.

There may be marked nervous excitement and prostration.

Headache better (>) cool air and motion until they become warmed up which then makes it worse (<); worse (<) lying down, warm wraps and noise. Throbbing, pressing bursting headache. Periodical headaches and headaches with stomach complaints. Often it is better (>) for eating and comes on if they miss a meal; headache with hunger.

Headache from suppressed nasal discharge, when a chronic, thick, yellow discharge is replaced by an acute, watery coryza with sneezing, then comes a headache which subsides when the thick, yellow discharge returns.

Thick, yellow, offensive ear discharges with loss of hearing and dry cough. Ear infections with eczema around and behind the ears.

Colds may settle in the nose and usually go to the chest with much whistling, wheezing and dyspnoea, worse (<) exertion. A dry teasing cough. Throbbing, burning and tickling in the chest.

Sore throats better for warm drinks, especially if they go from the right to the left side.

Cold extremities and a hot head; they want the head uncovered because of the congestion.

Great flatulence and belching is another marked symptom of this remedy. Everything eaten turns to wind and they may feel **full and distended after only a very few mouthfuls** with momentary relief (>) from belching. Gnawing pains and burning with gastritis and ulcers. Pains worse (<) cold drinks and better (>) warm drinks. Noisy rumbling. Diarrhoea of all kinds. They may desire sweets very much.

The urine may contain red sand or gravel. A headache may come on after the gravel stops coming out in the urine. They may be irritable on waking too.

Mercurius

- Sensitive to both heat and cold
- Offensive odours, of breath, sweat, discharges, stools, etc.
- Glands affected; inflamed and swollen
- Ulcerations of mucous membranes
- A tendency to suppuration

Sensitive to both heat and cold or open air, thus they have great difficulty in getting comfortable.

Offensive odours, of breath, sweat, discharges, stools etc.

Worse (<) night; pains in joints or inflammations which indurate. Worse (<) in the warmth of the bed.

Gland affected; inflamed and swollen.

Ulcerations; of mucous membranes.

Tendency to suppuration; it comes on rapidly with burning and stinging (like in *Apis*).

Catarrhs of mucous membranes; discharges start thin and excoriating and later become more thick and bland.

Rheumatic complaints.

Complaints with **sweating which is offensive, may be profuse but does not give relief (>)** and may even make them worse (<), (unlike *Arsenicum* and *Natrum mur.*).

Copious salivation; often with a **metallic taste** or sweet or salty and a sense of dryness with intense thirst sometimes.

Trembling.

Mercurius (continued)

- Catarrhs of mucous membranes
- Copious salivation; often with a metallic taste
- Tongue may be swollen, flabby, spongy, taking the imprint of the teeth
- Tenesmus with diarrhoea

Delirium in an acute illness. Many complaints are worse (<) lying on the right side.

Repeated swellings and abscess formation without any heat, they sweat all over and slowly emaciate, it keeps on discharging with no tendency to heal.

In a child after scarlet fever or a suppressed ear discharge with sweating of the head, dilated pupils, rolling of the head, worse (<) at night, in such lingering febrile conditions *Mercurius* may be needed.

In fevers they are chilly before the chill, a creeping chilliness in the evening which may increase into the night; very sensitive to a draught; cold hands and feet; profuse and offensive sweat which often makes things worse (<). Fevers are not as high as in *Belladonna*. Chilliness may alternate with flashes of heat like in *Arsenicum*.

In chronic catarrh with a thick discharge suppressed, possibly by a cold, and on comes a severe headache, in the forehead, face, ears. Much heat in the head with all the headaches; bursting, constricting pains.

Eye catarrh worse (<) sitting by the fire; every cold settles in the eyes in rheumatic patients. Colds may also go to the chest and linger.

Ears and nose produce a horrible, stinking, green discharge; ear infection with rupture and suppuration.

The tongue may be **swollen, flabby, spongy, taking the imprint of the teeth**, coated, foul with copious saliva and nothing tastes right. Gums may be swollen, spongy and bleeding.

Sore throat may have a swollen, spongy appearance, with flat spreading ulcers; sensation of great dryness. Difficulty swallowing from the pain and paralytic weakness. Quinsy.

Sour stomach with wind, regurgitation, reflux, nausea, food sitting like a load, the characteristic taste and salivation. Milk disagrees and comes up sour.

Tenesmus with diarrhoea.

Affects the right lower chest with stitches through to the back (like in *Kali carb.*).

Almost everything will make them worse (<) and virtually nothing will bring relief (>).

Natrum muriaticum

- Complaints following a loss, a grief, a rejection, unrequited love or a reprimand
- Often worse (<) 10–11 am
- Discharge from mucous membranes is watery or thick like white of egg
- Awful bursting headaches

Complaints following a loss, a grief, a rejection, unrequited love or a reprimand. They hold their feelings in, their grief, anger, frustration and would rarely weep in front of others. They may be sensitive to a change of weather.

There may be weakness, nervous prostration, nervous irritability and they desire solitude when they are ill; consolation makes worse (<). Greatly disturbed by excitement and they can be extremely emotional. The whole nervous economy may be in a state of fret and irritation; worse (<) sudden noises, may feel weak and ill afterwards, worse (<) music. Oversensitive and easily offended.

Worse (<) 10–11 am. Worse (<) lying down.

Pains are stitching, electric shock like, shooting with twitchings, jerkings and trembling.

They take cold easily when sweating or in a draught but are in general better (>) in the open air, though worse (<) on getting heated. They may usually be quite warm blooded people.

Natrum muriaticum (continued)

- Often worse (<) 10–11 am
- Thirst for cold drinks throughout
- Mucous membranes are dry

Discharge from mucous membranes is watery or thick like white of egg; from ears and eyes too.

Awful headaches; **bursting** compressing as if in a vice, as if would be crushed; hammering and throbbing pains; pains in the morning on waking. Great nervousness. They fall asleep late and wake with a headache. **Headache at 10 or 11 am**. Periodical headaches.

A bursting headache during the chill and fever with copious thirst and relief (>) during the sweat; other headaches are not relieved (>) by the sweat.

Headache from the inability to focus the eyes rapidly enough, from eye strain. Headache with sore eyes.

Chill at 10 or 11 am; starting in the extremities, with a throbbing head and flushed face. **Thirst for cold drinks throughout**. During the coldness they are not better (>) by heat or covering up and they still want **cold drinks despite chattering teeth** and aching bones; tossing and turning. In the fever there may be intense heat and they go into a congestive stupor or sleep. They may be delirious with constant talking and mania. The sweat ameliorates (>) sometimes everything except the headache.

Mucous membranes are dry; lips dry and cracked, split in the centre of the lips, cold sore on the lips, throat dry, red, patulous with a splinter sensation. Chronic dryness without ulceration. Much catarrhal discharge with dryness at other times; there may be a sense of dryness without actual dryness like in *Mercurius*. A bitter taste at times.

Slow digestion, sensation of a lump in the stomach after eating which disagrees (<). Bowels distended with gas. Stool hard and difficult. Stitching, tearing pains in the liver with fullness.

Cough from tickling low down, with bursting pain in the forehead. Stitches all over the chest.

Nux vomica

- Complaints coming from overindulgence in food, drink, spicy foods, stimulants of all sorts or from mental overwork
- Problems following exposure to cold dry winds
- Digestive upset
- Marked oversensitivity
- Severe chills in a fever

Complaints coming from overindulgence in food, drink, spicy foods, stimulants of all sorts or from mental overwork. Problems following exposure to cold dry winds.

The complaints are often accompanied by some sort of **digestive upset** (like in *Pulsatilla*).

Marked oversensitivity; irritable and touchy, never contented, never satisfied. They may be prone to arguments and quarrel over any imagined offence. They can feel hurried and driven, critical and quick to reproach. They may prefer to be left alone and hate having to depend on others who are less capable than themselves. They cannot stand contradiction and indeed they are often right. Even to being impulsive, an uncontrolled state of irritability; it is a weakness and is accompanied by physical weakness. They may be sleepless from an overactive mind and sensitivity to slight noises which disturb them. Feel as if they could fly to pieces. Weakness, twitching, trembling. This mental state may indicate the remedy on its own, like the emotional state of *Chamomilla* often does but there may be none of it apparent and yet the physical symptoms would still indicate its use.

A chilly person, sensitive to draughts. Sweats easily. Always taking cold which settles in the nose, throat or ears and goes to the chest. A warm room makes the coryza worse (<) before the fever comes on; after

Nux vomica (continued)

- When vomiting there is much retching, gagging and straining
- Much straining but only scanty stool
- Worse (<) eating
- Worse (<) cold

the fever they must have heat. **Severe chills in a fever**, they cannot get warm and cannot bear to uncover, which sends waves of chills through them. The heat is short and dry followed by intense heat and hot sweat worse (<) in the morning. A very red face in the fever.

Neuralgic headaches; stick and tear, burn and sting; drawing pains especially; a sensation of tension in the muscles.

Headache worse (<) mental exertion, anger, open air, on waking, after eating, coffee, spirits, sun, light, noise, stooping, movement, stormy weather. Headache with constipation and a sour stomach.

They may have a weak digestion and be intolerant of many foods yet crave pungent, bitter, spicy things, tonics or milk. Meat can cause nausea.

When vomiting there is **much retching, gagging and straining** before they can finally vomit. Likewise there may be **much strain-ing but only scanty stool**. The spasmodic, colicky abdominal pains are worse (<) motion and better (>) heat. *Nux* is **worse (<) eating** and suffers from dyspepsia, heartburn, neausea, fullness, constipation, bloating and gas. A feeling of pressure 1 or 2 hours after eating, like a stone even (*Bryonia, Pulsatilla* etc.). *Nux* is definitely **better (>) with an empty stomach**.

Backache worse (<) lying down, must get up and walk.

Dry teasing cough with great soreness of the chest. Spasmodic cough with retching; worse (<) cold dry windy weather. Tickling and pain in the larynx with the cough. Cough causes a bursting headache.

Worse (<) cold, uncovering, cold dry weather, eating and especially overeating stimulants, mornings, anger, mental exertion.

Better (>) evenings, resting, wet weather, after stool.

Phosphorus

- Sensitive to external stimuli; odours, touch, noise, cold etc
- Flushes of heat
- Haemorrhages
- Headaches are congestive and throbbing
- Hunger
- Violent thirst for ice cold and refreshing drinks
- Vomiting of warm drinks
- Hoarseness worse (<) in evening

Complaints may come on from electric changes in the atmosphere.

Flushes of heat. Often in people subject to violent pulsations, palpitations and congestions.

Haemorrhages; anaemia and relaxed conditions of muscles.

Burning pains, tearing and drawing pains. Sensation of intense heat running up the back.

May be very sensitive to all external stimuli; odours, touch noise, cold etc. which can lead to exhaustion. Always tired and want to rest. Great prostration of mind or body after mental or physical effort. Weakness to paralysis even. Trembling from slight causes; great excitability, can be restless and fidgety. May want to be rubbed, massaged. Full of anxieties and fears but usually easily reassured.

Vertigo and dizziness is common.

Headaches are congestive and throbbing; blood mounts to the head; better (>) cold and rest, worse (<) heat, motion and lying down; often they have to sit up and apply pressure to the head and a cold application. Face flushed and hot. **Hunger** can precede or accompany the headaches.

Coryza; painful dryness in the nose; sneezing and running of the nose may be with blood. Yellow, green discharges too.

Phosphorus (continued)

- Oppression and constriction in the chest
- Flushes of blood and heat going upwards in the chest

Swollen glands in weak, sickly, pale, exhausted people.

Violent thirst for ice cold, and refreshing drinks; dry mouth and throat. Sore, excoriated, bleeding mouth. Swollen tonsils; dysphagia and constriction.

Hunger may be violent; must eat during the chill, at night, with the headache. Must eat or they will faint; hungry empty feeling in the whole abdomen.

Vomiting of warm drinks in stomach upset. They may desire cold food, sour, spicy things, wine.

Laryngitis with **hoarseness worse (<) in the evening**; larynx so painful they cannot talk; very sensitive to touch and cold air. Violent tickling in the larynx and behind the sternum. Colds may go to the larynx from every change of weather.

A hard, dry, rasping cough, exhausting; so painful that they suppress the cough.

Anxiety, weakness, **oppression and constriction** in the chest; sensation as if a great weight were on the chest. Tightness. **Flushes of blood and heat going upwards in the chest**. Painful chest especially in the right lower zone, better (>) for pressure. Blood stained sputum, salty, sour or yellow. Suffocation and constriction better (>) pressure. Bursting headache with the cough. Cough worse (<) open air, **going from a warm to a cold room** or vice versa, twilight, lying on left side, talking, eating; better (>) lying on right side.

Violent palpitations worse (<) lying on left side, motion. May sleep on right side for preference.

Stiffness on beginning to move in the morning.

Worse (<) cold weather.

Better (>) heat except stomach and head, rest.

Pulsatilla

- A gentle, mild, yielding person desiring attention
- Changeable in mood
- Clingy, whiny child who evokes your sympathy
- Desires company and comforting which ameliorates
- Worse (<) heat, they desire cool, open air
- Flushes to the face
- Better (>) slow gentle motion
- Thirstlessness

This remedy is often selected on its emotional picture:

A gentle, mild, yielding person **desiring attention**. Nervous, fidgety, **changeable in mood**, easily led. **A clingy, whiny child who evokes your sympathy**. May be fussy and irritable but not like the trantrums of *Chamomilla* or the touchiness of *Hepar*. **Desires company and comforting which ameliorates** (>). Moods may change easily from laughter to sadness; they cry easily even at the thought of pain. They tend to be sweet and loving when well but self-pitying when ill. Indecisive. They may not look ill.

Complaints may follow getting the feet wet; dietary indulgence especially of rich foods which upset them.

Worse (<) **heat is marked, they desire cool open air**. The skin feels hot even without a fever. **Flushes to the face**.

Better (>) slow gentle motion; this soothes them both generally and their specific complaints – pains, headaches etc.

Thirstlessness is usual even with a fever or the **dry mouth** which is also commonly present.

Changeability is marked even on the physical level; diarrhoea with no two stools alike; their pains may wander and symptoms change. Pains can come on suddenly and be slow to disappear.

Catarrhs of any mucous membrane which is inflamed and can look purplish, are common. The discharges are **thick, yellow/green**

Pulsatilla (continued)

- Changeability is marked
- Catararrhs thick, yellow/green and bland
- Digestive complaints often accompany every illness
- Worse (<) rich and fatty foods
- Digestive complaints worse (<) morning, mental complaints worse (<) evening
- One sided complaints
- Many eye, ear and nose catarrhal complaints

and bland. With nasal catarrh of some duration there may be loss of smell or taste.

Digestive complaints often accompany every illness; bloated and sensitive especially worse (<) after eating. Prefers cold things and is **worse (<) rich and fatty foods**, ice cream, pork, fruit, cold things; they may crave the foods which make them worse (<). **Tongue coated**, bad taste in the mouth especially early in the morning.

Digestive complaints are worse (<) in the morning and mental complaints are worse (<) **worse in the evening**.

Also worse (<) **at rest**; becomes frantic. Better (>) lying on the painful side. May not be able to sleep on the left side because of the palpitations and suffocation.

One sided complaints; fever, headache, sweat, chill etc.

Headache throbbing, congestive and is better (>) cold, pressure, tying the head up tightly, slow motion and worse (<) evening and stooping. Pains in the temples and sides

often. Headaches before menses which are often scanty.

Many eye, ear and nose catarrhal complaints. Itching eyelids; styes are better (>) cold, worse (<) heat with the typical discharge. The nose stuffs up in the evening and in a warm room. It is stuffed up on rising but they can clear it out. Nosebleeds are common.

Chills begin in the hands and feet with pains in the limbs; one sided; numbness; fever. Thirst before the chill. Profuse sweat all over or on one side. Heat with distended blood vessels. Vomiting of mucus in the chill at times.

Pains accompanied by constant chilliness and the more the pains the worse the chilliness.

Dry cough at night worse (<) lying down and a loose cough in the morning. Thick yellow green mucus.

Cough from tickling in the larynx; dry and teasing, wants fresh air. Coughs from inspiration; worse (<) evening and warm room.

Rhus toxicodendron

- Affects the joints, ligaments, tendons and skin
- Complaints come on from cold and damp weather or exposure, getting the feet wet or exposure whilst perspiring, overexertion, strained muscles
- Worse (<) cold
- Better (>) heat and motion

This remedy particularly affects the joints, ligaments, tendons and skin.

Complaints come on from **cold and damp weather or exposure, getting the feet wet or exposure whilst perspiring, overexertion, strained muscles**. Complaints often start at night.

Worse (<) cold in all complaints, worse (<) uncovering, evening and night, overexertion, getting wet.

Better (>) **heat and motion** (like *Pulsatilla*) but *Rhus* wants it warm, better (>) pressure, rubbing, perspiration.

First motion makes them worse (<)but continued motion ameliorates (>) but then on

comes exhaustion and they have to stop and **rest which makes them worse (<)** again. Therefore they are never perfectly at ease and may toss and turn in bed.

Restless, anxious, **aching sore and bruised pains, tearing pains**. Pains often with numbness and weakness of the limbs. Prominent projections of the bones can become sore to touch, especially the cheek bones.

Fever type headaches; the brain feels loose, **stupefying** with buzzing in the ears. Sensation as if parts of the skull were screwed together. Sore muscles and sore skull. Occipital pain better (>) holding the head back; great restlessness with this and aching better

Rhus toxicodendron (continued)

- First motion makes them worse (<) but continued motion ameliorates (>)
- Restless, anxious
- Aching, sore and bruised pains, tearing pains
- Stupefying headaches
- Red, triangular tip to tongue
- Eruptions are red, itchy and often with blisters

(>) for motion. The side of the scalp on which they lie may be sensitive and headaches may be worse (<) for wetting the hair.

Low forms of fever, incoherent talking, answers hastily with anxiety and mild delirium all worse (<) at night. Mild, persistent delirium, not as violent as in *Belladonna*; restless with laborious dreams, muttering delirium.

Colds settle throughout the body and limbs. Full of dizziness. Violent coryza; nose stopped up from every coryza. Great soreness of the nostrils. The discharge can be yellow, green, thick, offensive.

Cold may go to the larynx producing hoarseness better (>) for using the voice, rawness and roughness. Sore throat with swollen glands and a stiff neck.

Thirst is usually marked but there can be dysphagia for solids from the constricton. Dry mucous membranes; dry or coated tongue with a **red triangular tip**. Cold drinks can bring on chilliness or cough.

Dry, teasing, tickling cough before or during the chill; racking cough. Cough during sleep; cough from the least uncovering. Pneumonia or pleurisy with sharp, stitching pains in the chest, much fever, aching bones, restlessness and generally better (>) motion but prostration comes on, marked thirst and fever. Fevers with cold sores on the lips.

Hungry sensation without appetite sometimes.

Stiff lame back, better (>) lying on a hard floor; sore joints and tearing pains down the limbs.

Eruptions are red, itchy and often with blisters. Urticaria during heat.

Rumex

- The respiratory symptoms are its main indication for use
- A hoarse, barking cough in attacks every night at 11 pm, at 2 and 5 am
- Cough from the slightest breathing of cold air
- Cough worse (<) lying down
- Very sensitive to cold air
- Sit without motion

It does not have the febrile symptoms of *Bryonia*, *Rhus tox.* and *Aconite*, nor does it have the general disturbance; the aching limbs, the general soreness, the fever and thirst.

The **respiratory symptoms are its main indication for use**.

A hoarse, barking cough in attacks **every night at 11 pm, at 2 and 5 am**. Cough with pain behind the midsternum. **Cough worse (<) lying down** which causes the most violent cough to appear a few moments later. **Cough from the slightest breathing of cold air**, like *Phosphorus* and *Spongia*, from going from warm to cold. **Very sensitive to cold air**, must cover their mouths to protect from the cold air.

Copious, thin, frothy, white mucus is coughed up by the mouthful. There may also be a hard, dry, spasmodic cough at first. Watery expectoration that later becomes thick, yellow, stringy and tenacious. This often accompanies a brown, morning diarrhoea. Cough with the loss of a little urine, (like *Causticum*).

Extreme rawness in the larynx and trachea, burning and smarting. They cannot endure any pressure on the pit of the throat. Tickling in the pit of the throat or down the centre of the chest to the stomach, causes

Rumex (continued)

coughing and may be with a congested head and wrenching pains in the right of the chest.

Sit without motion, they cannot breathe deeply or rapidly because the burning is increased so much by any change in the pattern of respiration. Cough from changes of temperature.

Lachesis children cough in their early sleep at about 11 pm but if kept awake they will not cough. However in *Rumex* they will cough in either case.

Sensitive to open air and sometimes a sensation of breathlessness as if they were passing rapidly through the air.

Intense itching of the skin when undressing to go to bed may be present.

Silica

- Complaints after getting the feet wet from suppressed discharges or sweat
- Catarrhs; with a thick, yellow discharge
- Lymph nodes enlarge and become hard
- Worse (<) warm rooms and heat
- Sweat about the upper part of the body or head
- Headache from back of head going over forehead

Symptoms often come on in cold damp weather and may be improved by cold dry weather.

Complaints after getting the feet wet, (like *Pulsatilla*), from suppressed discharges or sweat. It is easily affected by extremes of temperature, easily overheats and sweats then takes cold.

Catarrhs; with a thick, yellow discharge.

Lymph nodes enlarge and become hard especially in the neck; inflamed glands.

Acute illnesses are **worse (<) warm rooms and heat**, whereas normally they are chilly and worse (<) draughts.

Sweat about the upper part of the body or head; offensive.

Headache from the back of the head going over the forehead worse (<) night, noise, cold air, better (>) heat and pressure. Headache with profuse head sweat.

Suppuration of lid margins with stinging, burning and redness. Photophobia is marked. Eyes inflamed from trauma or after foreign bodies have been removed.

Chronic ear discharges; offensive, thick, yellow; roaring and hissing in the ears; eustachian catarrh; the hearing returns with a snap, better (>) gaping or swallowing.

Hard crusts accumulate in the nose with loss of taste and smell. Nosebleeds.

Rough lips; they crack and peel, crusty at the margins of the mucous membranes or on the ears.

Nausea, vomiting and hiccup with aversion to warm food and desire for cold food. Hot drinks cause sweating and hot flushes in the face and head. Milk aggravates (<) and causes diarrhoea and vomiting; sour vomiting; sour curds in the stool. Colic and sore to pressure, worse (<) after eating and better (>) heat.

Spigelia

- Intense pains that are shooting, burning, stabbing, tearing, neuralgic
- Pains that increase as the sun rises to midday and decrease as it falls and sets
- Worse (<) motion
- Headaches are often one sided beginning in the occiput and extending forward and settling over the left eye

This remedy is known by its **pains**.

Pains from taking cold in run down persons.

There are shooting, burning, stabbing, tearing, neuralgic pains. **Intense pains**.

Pains that increase as the sun rises to midday and decrease as it falls and sets (like in *Natrum mur* and *Tabacum*).

Worse (<) motion; even mental exertion makes the pains worse (<).

Worse (<) eating, in the morning, noise, cold damp rainy weather.

Better (>) for quiet and dry air.

Pains in the neck and shoulders better (>) heat; cannot move because of pain

Pains about the eyes better (>) for cold.

Head pains are worse (<) heat and are temporarily better (>) from cold applications. Trigeminal neuralgia, especially of the left side.

Painful parts can become red, inflamed and sensitive. Pulsating and stitching pains in the head may be better (>) lying with the head held high, worse (<) motion, stooping, noise.

Pains in the extremities like hot wires usually better (>) keeping still; so sore that any jar is unbearable. Vertigo from looking downward, therefore they sit and look straight ahead.

Headaches are often one sided beginning in the occiput and extending forward and settling over the left eye (right is *Sanguinaria*, *Silica* etc.). The eye of the affected side may water with tears.

Spongia

- Similar to *Aconite* but lacks its febrile excitement and is slower in pace
- Worse (<) warm room and heat but better (>) for warm drinks
- Remedy for croup,
- Exposure to dry cold winds
- Roughness and dryness of the mucous membranes
- Dry/cough with no rattling

This remedy is similar to *Aconite* but lacks its febrile exicitement and is slower in pace, its onset taking several days and often beginning in the evening. It is another remedy with an affinity for the respiratory tract.

Mentally there may be marked anxiety even to fear of death and suffocation. Palpitations and uneasiness in the heart region; pain and a sense of fullness or stuffiness in the heart region or chest. They may wake from sleep with great fear, agitation and anxiety and a sense of suffocation like in *Lachesis*.

Worse (<) warm room and heat but is better (>) for warm drinks.

A main remedy for **croup**, especially if it follows taking cold or **exposure to dry cold winds** 1 or 2 days previously. First there appears a **roughness and dryness of the mucous membranes**, sneezing and croup comes on before midnight with a dry, hoarse, barking cough, like a saw being driven through a plank of wood, and **dry air passages**. The more rattling there is the more likely *Hepar sulph.* is to be indicated, especially if inclined to get worse after midnight or in the morning hours, and the less it is likely *Spongia* will be the remedy. **Dry with no rattling is *Spongia*** and it may follow *Aconite* if the croup continues after midnight and into the next day. Wake from sleep with suffocation, alarm, anxiety and a loud cough. Later tough mucus may form which is difficult to expectorate.

Dyspnoea is **worse (<) lying down**, with the head low, better (>) for warm food. Cough **better (>)** for **warm food and drink**, worse (<) talking, singing, swallowing, awakening from sleep.

Hoarseness with loss of voice, **great dryness of the larynx** from a cold; coryza, sneezing, the whole chest rings, is very dry; voice is hissy, croupy and dry.

After taking a cold, rawness of the larynx and trachea come on, then spasmodic constriction of the larynx at night. The larynx is sensitive to touch (like *Phosphorus*).

If the symptoms tend to relapse or get more croupy every evening, then *Phosphorus* may be indicated and should be studied.

Violent basilar headaches, worse (<) lying down, they must sit up and keep still.

In the laryngitis and bronchitis of adults it is as useful as in the croups of children (especially *Aconite* and *Hepar*). **Great hoarseness, some soreness and burning** and the **cough is worse (<) talking, reading, singing, swallowing**.

Cough worse (<) cold air, evening and morning, better (>) drinking and eating warm things.

This remedy may come up after a *Belladonna* sore throat has gone down on the chest.

Sulphur

- Healthy people who are emotionally thick skinned
- Burning – pains, eruptions, sensations and discharges
- Offensive odours – sweat, discharges
- Aversion to washing
- Very thirsty
- Heat on top of the head; feet burn at night in bed, hot flushes rising up. Congestions
- Worse (<) heat, standing, at night, 12 am or 12 pm
- Hunger at 11 am; feels faint and weak
- Catarrhs, especially lingering catarrhs

Often needed for robust, healthy people who are emotionally thick skinned.

Burning – pains, eruptions, sensations and discharges. The feet, eyes, ears, nose, throat, vertex of head, stomach, chest all **burn**.

Offensive odours – sweat, discharges; the patient himself may be unaware of the smell.

Aversion to washing and it can make the skin worse (<); worse (<) for water and bathing.

Very thirsty usually.

Heat on top of the head; feet burn at night in bed, hot flushes rising up. Congestions; they feel so oppressed that they want the window open, especially at night. **Worse (<) heat. Eruptions itch and burn. Warmth of the bed produces uneasiness.**

Worse (<) 12 am or 12 pm.

Worse (<) at night, with sinking and exhaustion.

Worse (<) standing, bathing. Better (>) sitting, lying.

Hunger at 11 am; feels faint and weak.

Catarrhs of all mucous membranes; suppurations with burning discharges; ulcerations; acrid discharges.

Burning, stinging, itching eruptions worse (<) heat. Inflammation from pressure and it can indurate. Skin affected easily by the atmosphere, becomes red from the wind and the cold; flushes begin in the chest and rise up; dusky red at the least provocation. Skin itching worse (<) for heat, scratching ameliorates (>) but it turns to burning.

Ruddy, purple appearance which may alternate with paleness plus the flushes of heat. Purplish throat, rash, a venous appearance.

Sleepless yet they are worse (<) if they oversleep; lethargic.

Diarrhoea which drives them from bed in the morning, worse (<) at 5 am.

Dyspnoea, especially on exertion, copious sweat and so exhausted. Rattling in the chest; every cold goes to the chest or nose **and the catarrh hangs on a long time**. The patient does not convalesce, complains that they are slow to pick up, cannot muster the energy to get better. Lingering cough after a chest infection. Problems that improve temporarily and then relapse again and the previously effective remedy no longer works; a dose or two of *Sulphur* in this situation will often either clear up the problem or will allow the indicated remedy to work again.

Red lips, eyelids and around the orifices of the body.

A violent racking cough in bronchitis. Suffocating and wants doors and windows open at night. Night cough. Cough with congested head. Burning in the chest etc.

A remedy commonly needed in measles, especially if the rash has not come out fully or has disappeared again and they become more ill.

They may be impatient, hurried and quick tempered in an acute illness.

Appendix

§23 Conditions requiring constitutional therapy

Chronic diseases reflect the state of health at a much deeper level than the simple acute illnesses whose treatment is outlined in this book. They are by their very nature more complex, particularly in the Western world where health disorders often reflect the complexity of our lifestyles and the variety of stresses we experience. It is not uncommon to find the pattern of health changing every few years in response to a stressful environment. For example, as a child someone may experience only colds and sore throats, in their teens headaches may occur, their twenties may bring abdominal pains, and in their thirties a diagnosis of Irritable Bowel Syndrome is made. This sequence of events, if unchanged, could progress to other more serious conditions. At each stage the person is becoming more ill and, although the previous 'disease' disappeared, it was not cured. It merely changed its form and became manifest in a different area. Looked at as a whole it can be seen to be the same 'disease' throughout life.

Whilst chronic conditions require full constitutional treatment they often have an acute element. For instance an arthritis may flare up in a particular joint for a few days or a hiatus hernia may cause acute heartburn or vomiting. This acute element is even more apparent in recurrent illness such as migraine, hay fever or period pains. The acute episodes of such illnesses can be treated in a manner similar to simple acute illnesses. It may well be possible to use this book to find remedies that will give relief from whatever pain or discomfort each time it occurs but, as was said at the end of Chapter 1, it will not prevent the pain from recurring next time.

The curative treatment of chronic and recurrent conditions (see Table 1) is, for the reasons stated above, beyond the scope of this book and has been deliberately omitted.

Table of some of the common disorders *not* covered by this book.

Allergic disorders	Haemorrhoids (piles)	**Peptic ulceration**
Arthritis	**Hiatus hernia**	Pre-menstrual syndrome
Asthma	**Irritable bowel syndrome**	Raynaud's phenomenon
Athlete's foot	Leg ulcers	Ringworm
Bronchitis	Menstrual irregularity	Shingles
Eczema	**Migraines**	Squint
Endometriosis	M.E.	Tinnitus
Glandular fever	Nasal polyps	Verruca
Glue ear	Parasitic infections	Warts

Those printed in bold type have acute episodes. They can often be helped with remedies which can be found from the information in this book.
An exhaustive list would run on for many pages. If in doubt about a particular condition, consult your health care practitioner.

§24 Sources of information

Homoeopathy: professional associations

British Homoeopathic Association.
27a Devonshire Street,
London W1N 1RJ.
Tel: 071 935 2163

Society of Homoeopaths.
2 Artizan Road,
Northampton NN1 4HU.
Tel: 0604 21400

These organisations will supply lists of registered practitioners.

Homoeopathy: training colleges

Faculty of Homoeopathy.
Royal London Homoeopathic Hospital,
Great Ormond Street,
London WC1N 3HR.
Tel: 071 837 3091 ext 72

Midlands College of Homoeopathy.
186 Wolverhampton Street,
Dudley,
West Midlands DY1 3AD.

College of Homoeopathy.
26 Clarendon Rise,
London SE13 6JR.
Tel: 081 852 0573

London College of Classical
Homoeopathy.
63 Maycross Avenue,
Morden, Surrey.
Tel: 081 540 6041

Northern College of Homoeopathic
Medicine.
114a High Street,
Gosforth,
Newcastle upon Tyne NE3 1HB.
Tel: 091 284 8010

The Small School of Homoeopathy.
Out of the Blue Centre,
North Street,
Cromford,
Derbyshire DE4 3RG.
Tel: 0629 824574

The number of colleges is increasing rapidly.
A full list is available from the Society of Homoeopaths. Most courses are part time and do not require previous medical training.

Holistic medicine

The Natural Medicines Society.
Edith Lewis House,
Back Lane,
Ilkeston,
Derbyshire DE7 8EJ.
Tel: 0636 329454

This society was formed to protect and develop natural and holistic medicine. At the time of writing it is particularly concerned to ensure that legislation on the assessment of natural medical products is appropriate to the therapies using those medicines. The assessments used for orthodox medicines are totally inappropriate for those of Homoeopathic and herbal medicine.

The Natural Medicines Society has formed a committee of experts who will be able to advise the legislators in such a way that the law can be properly formulated in relation to the alternative therapies. Support from the professions and the public is needed to enable their voice to be heard where it matters. The society is a registered charity.

Useful addresses:

Ainsworths Homoeopathic Pharmacy.
38 New Cavendish Street,
London W1M 7LH.
Tel: 071 935 5330

Galen Homoeopathics.
Lewell Mill,
West Stafford,
Dorchester,
Dorset DT2 8AN.
Tel: 0305 63996

Foresight.
The Old Vicarage,
Church Lane,
Witley,
Near Godalming,
Surrey GU8 5PN.

Helios Homoeopathic Pharmacy.
92 Camden Road,
Tunbridge Wells,
Kent TN1 2QP.
Tel: 0892 36393

Weleda (UK) Ltd.
Heanor Road,
Ilkeston,
Derbyshire DE7 8DR.
Tel: 0602 309319

Pakua lotion and cream are obtainable from:
M & HS Co.
Curwood House,
Kent's Close,
Uffculme,
Devon EX13 3AW.

§25 Remedies and pharmacies

How can I be sure of the quality of the remedies on sale?

The simplest answer to that question is 'You cannot, unless you make the remedies yourself!' Not to worry! When buying remedies there are several things to look for which will indicate a high quality product. Ask your local or usual supplier.

How are the remedies themselves actually prepared? Are they succussed by hand or by machine? Succussion is part of the process of potentising a remedy which involves vigorous shaking (succussion) and a series of dilutions. In the author's opinion, the most important change in this process is not the material one of dilution but is concerned with the change in energy, vital force, chi, consciousness or whatever else you may be used to calling it. At any rate, practical experience teaches that the most 'potent' remedies are prepared by hand. Those prepared by mechanical succussion tend to be less effective. This is, therefore, the single most important question to ask.

What are the circumstances in which the remedies are prepared? Are they prepared quietly, calmly, methodically by someone paying attention to what they are doing? For similar reasons to those just given, the greater the attention and awareness of the person preparing the remedy, the more active will the end product be.

What safeguards are taken to ensure that one remedy does not, by its dust or vapour, contaminate another remedy in the preparation process?

Are the raw ingredients of the highest quality? For instance, with remedies prepared from plants, are they picked at the best time of the year, the best time of the day and in the best weather conditions to produce a high quality plant tincture from which to prepare the remedy? All the specific conditions for growing, picking and preparing remedies are described precisely in the various homoeopathic pharmacopoeia used by the pharmacist.

How much care is taken to ensure that the remedies are not handled?

Are they stored away from direct sunlight (which inactivates remedies) and preferably in secure, glass bottles?

It is not always the largest manufacturers who take the greatest care in preparing potentised remedies. Some do but often you will find that remedies prepared by small homoeopathic pharmacies are much more potent.

Of the large manufacturers, the author uses products from Weleda and of the pharmacies he uses Helios Homoeopathic Pharmacy in Tunbridge Wells, Kent and The Galen Pharmacy in Dorchester, Dorset. There will be many other excellent sources, of which the author has no experience. Most will accept telephone orders which, if given early enough in the day, will frequently be dispatched on the same day. Large orders may take a little longer. See the list of addresses at the end of the previous section.

We now come to another question:

Which remedies do I need to buy?

This is really an impossible one to answer because each person's health demands are different. However in the author's opinion the most basic kit should contain at least 24 remedies in one potency. This may be thought, by some beginners, to be too many to start with, so 12 of the most commonly required remedies have been suggested as a starter kit. More comprehensive kits containing a further 24 remedies each time, are also suggested up to a total of 72. On the assumption that you already possess the basic 24 remedies, a few additional remedies are suggested to meet specific needs. Most of the additional remedies are amongst the total of 72. The question of potency is dealt with in the section on how to use the book. The 12c potency was recommended but the suitable range is from a 6x to a 30c.

Starter kit of 12 remedies. *Aconite, Apis, Arnica, Belladonna, Bryonia, Chamomilla, Ferrum phosphoricum, Gelsemium, Ipecacuanha, Pulsatilla, Rhus toxicodendron, Sulphur.*

A useful addition to the kit would be some *Calendula* ointment or tincture, which can be diluted in water 1 in 25 to bathe, clean and dress cuts, scrapes, wounds, burns, ulcers etc.

Basic kit (includes all the remedies in the starter kit and 12 more). *Aconite, Allium cepa, Apis, Arnica, Arsenicum, Belladonna, Bryonia, Chamomilla, Colocynthis, Dioscorea, Euphrasia, Ferrum phosphoricum, Gelsemium, Hepar sulphuris, Hypericum, Ipecacuanha, Ledum, Lycopodium, Magnesia phosphorica, Mercurius, Nux vomica, Pulsatilla, Rhus toxicodendron, Sulphur.*

Intermediate kit (additional 24 remedies). *Antimonium tartaricum, Argentum nitricum, Bellis perennis, Calcarea carbonica, Causticum, Drosera, Dulcamara, Eupatorium perfoliatum, Jaborandi, Kali bichromicum, Lac caninum, Lachesis, Natrum muriaticum, Nitric acid, Phosphorus, Phytolacca, Podophyllum, Pyrogen, Ruta, Sanguinaria, Silica, Spigelia, Spongia, Urtica urens.*

Comprehensive kit (final 24 remedies). *Antimonium crudum, Baptisia, Calcarea phosphorica, Camphor, Carbo vegetabilis, Cantharis, China, Cocculus, Coffea, Cuprum, Glonoin, Hyoscyamus, Ignatia, Iris, Kali carbonicum, Kreosotum, Mercurius cyanatus, Natrum sulphuricum, Petroleum, Rumex, Staphisagria, Sepia, Symphytum, Tabacum, Veratum album.*

Additions to the basic kit

Measels, mumps and chicken pox. *Antimonium tartaricum, Camphor, Carbo vegetabilis, Jaborandi, Kali bichromicum, Phytolacca.*

Travel sickness. *Cocculus, Petroleum, Sepia, Staphisagria, Tabacum.*

First aid. *Bellis perennis, Calcarea phosphorica, Cantharis, Causticum, Cuprum, Eupatorium perfoliatum, Glonoin, Lachesis, Natrum muriaticum, Phosphorus, Silica, Staphisagria, Symphytum, Urtica urens.*

Diarrhoea and vomiting. *Antimonium crudum, Antimonium tartaricum, Carbo vegetabilis, China, Dulcamara, Natrum sulphuricum, Phosphorus, Podophyllum, Sepia, Veratrum album.*

Cystitis. *Cantharis, Causticum, Kali muriaticum, Kali phosphoricum, Natrum muriaticum, Sarsaparilla, Staphisagria.*

Period pains. *Calcarea fluorica, Calcarea phosphorica, Cocculus, Conium, Kali phosphoricum, Lachesis, Sepia*

Vaginal thrush. *Candida, Kali muriaticum Sepia.*

Remedies for mother and baby

Birthing. *Aconite M, Arnica 200, Bellis Perennis M, Caulophyllum 10M, Ipecacuanha 200, Kali phosphoricum 12x, Pulsatilla 200.* Rescue remedy (Bach flowers) also useful.

Breast feeding. *Castor equi 3x, Hydrastis 6x or 12, Phytolacca 6x or 12.*

Mastitis. *Belladonna *, Bryonia*, Hepar sulphuris *, Mercurius *, Phytolacca.*

Milk supply. *Calcarea carbonica, Lac defloratum, Pulsatilla *.*

After Pains. *Arnica *, Conium.*

Baby colic. *Chamomilla *, Colocynthis *, Dioscorea *, Magnesia phosphorica *.*

(* in basic kit).

These are suggestions to help the beginner get started. You may find that your family, or whoever you treat, will tend to have more of one type of illness than another and you will need to expand your remedy kit with remedies particularly suited to that type of condition. Be flexible in your approach and see what you need; never mind what I (or any one else) tell you!

Further reading

Home prescribing guides

There are many guides to choose from reflecting the different approaches to Homoeopathy and the levels to which it can be studied. I have attempted to arrange the following selection of books in order of increasing depth and complexity, though very often the style and layout are of far greater importance. A beginner might get on with one of the books at the end of the list even though it provides far more information.

Homoeopathy for the Family
  The Homoeopathic Development Foundation.

Homoeopathic Treatment for Children
  Phylis Speight

Homoeopathic Medicine at Home
  Panos, Maesimund and Heimlich TARCHER

Homoeopathy for the First Aider
  Dorothy Shepherd HEALTH SCIENCE PRESS

First Aid Homoeopathy in Accidents and Ailments
  D. M. Gibson BRITISH HOMOEOPATHIC ASSOCIATION

Homoeopathic Medicine: A Doctor's Guide to Remedies for Common Ailments
  Trevor Smith THORSONS

Everybody's Guide to Homoeopathic Medicines
  Cummings and Ullman TARCHER

The Complete Homoeopathy Handbook
  Miranda Castro MACMILLAN

Homoeopathy

The books listed here are not home prescribing guides. The first is a very good general introduction to Homoeopathy. The rest take the subject further and provide stimulating reading.

Homoeopathy. Medicine of the New Man
  George Vithoulkas THORSONS

The Challenge of Homoeopathy
  Margery Blackie UNWIN HYMAN

Homoeopathic Medicine
  Harris Coulter FORMUR

Homoeopathy in Epidemic Diseases
Magic of the Minimum Dose
More Magic of the Minimum Dose
A Physician's Posy
  Dorothy Shepherd
  HEALTH SCIENCE PRESS

The Science of Homoeopathy
  George Vithoulkas THORSONS

Glossary

Abdomen: part of body lying between chest and pelvis.

Abscess: localised collection of pus caused by suppuration in a tissue, organ or confined space.

Acrid: irritating, excoriating, bitter.

Acute: of sudden onset and brief duration.

-algia (suffix): 'pain in . . .' for example arthralgia = pain in joints.

Basilar headache: headache at base of head.

Bilious: containing bile (bitter, dark yellow/green pigments).

Blepharitis: inflammation of eye lid margins.

Candida: *Candida albicans*, fungus affecting mucous membranes and skin. Causes thrush.

Carotid artery: one of the main pairs of arteries in the front of the neck supplying head.

Catarrh: discharge of mucus from inflamed mucous membranes.

Chicken pox: acute infectious disease caused by a virus, with malaise, fever and characteristic rash (red elevated vesicles or blisters which crust over and come in crops).

Chronic: persisting for a long time, a state showing no change or very slow change over a long period.

Coccyx: little bone at base or tail end of spine.

Colic: acute abdominal pain that gradually increases and then decreases in an intermittent manner, usually lasting for a few minutes each time.

Concussion: violent shock or blow to brain; may cause vertigo, nausea, loss of consciousness.

Concomitant: a symptom coming at the same time as but not directly related to the main complaint.

Congestion: abnormal accumulation of blood in a part.

Constipation: abnormally infrequent or difficult bowel movements.

Cornea: transparent front part of eye.

Coryza: profuse discharge from mucous membranes of nose – 'common cold'.

Cramp: painful spasmodic muscular contraction.

Croup: inflammatory condition of larynx and trachea, usually of children, with laryngeal spasm, breathlessness and difficult, noisy breathing.

Cystitis: inflammation of the bladder.

Delirium: a confused excited state marked by incoherent speech, illusion, hallucinations and disorientation.

Diarrhoea: frequent evacuation of loose (watery) stools.

Discharge: an excretion or substance evacuated from the body.

Dysentery: inflammation of large intestine with evacuation of liquid and bloody stools and tenesmus.

Dyspepsia: indigestion.

Dysphagia: difficulty swallowing.

Dyspnoea: laboured or difficult breathing.

Eczema: an inflammatory disease of skin with redness, itching, soreness and sometimes discharging vesicles.

Emaciation: wasted, lean body.

Engorged: excessive fullness of any organ.

Episiotomy: cutting the vulva to faclitate childbirth.

Eructations: oral ejection of gas or air from stomach (belching).

Eruption: skin lesions or rash (not due to external injury).

Eustachian tube: canal from middle ear to back of throat (nasopharynx).

Excoriate: remove an area of skin.

Expectorate: to eject phelgm from air passages.

Exudate: inflammatory material deposited in tissues or oozed out on tissue surfaces from ulcers etc.

Faeces: excrement, stools.

Febrile: feverish.

Fever: elevation of body temperature above normal 36.8°C (98.4°F).

Fibrous tissue: common connective tissue of body.

Foetid: having a rank, disagreeable smell.

Flatus (flatulent): gas or air in stomach or intestines; wind coming up or going down!

Follicular: pouch-like depression.

Frontal headache: headache across forehead.

Gastritis: inflammation of stomach.

Genitalia: organs of reproduction.

Generals: symptoms relating to the whole person that can be expressed 'I am . . .' (compare with 'Particulars').

Glands: refers to lymph nodes unless otherwise stated.

Haemorrhage: escape of blood from a ruptured blood vessel.

Haemorrhoids: piles, anal varicose veins.

Hawking: forceful coughing up of phlegm from throat.

Hyperaesthesia: sensations abnormally increased.

Hyperventilation: abnormally deep, rapid or prolonged breathing.

Induration: abnormally hardened area.

Infection: multiplication of pathogenic (disease producing) micro-organisms within the body.

Inflammation: protective tissue response to injury or destruction of body cells characterised by heat, swelling, redness and usually pain.

Iris: circular coloured part of eye.

Iritis: inflammation of iris.

-itis (suffix): 'inflammation of ...' for example arthritis = inflammation of joints.

Jaundice: yellowness of skin and eyes from bile pigments.

Laceration: wound, torn flesh.

Lardaceous: having the appearance of lard; a fatty, greasy appearance.

Larynx: part of the top of wind-pipe containing vocal cords.

Laryngitis: inflammation of larynx.

Lassitude: weariness and disinclination to exert or interest oneself.

Ligaments: band of tough fibrous tissue connecting two bones at a joint (or supporting an organ of the body).

Loquacious: excessively talkative.

Lymph nodes: small masses of specialised tissue at intervals in lymphatic system for filtering off foreign particles; can often be felt in neck, arm pits, groins, etc. especially when enlarged through disease.

Malaise: feeling of unease, discomfort or being unwell.

Mania: mental derangement marked by excitement, hyperactivity, hallucination and sometimes violence.

Mastitis: inflammation of the breast.

Materia medica: branch of science dealing with the origins and properties of remedies.

Measles: acute, infectious disease caused by a virus characterised by a fever, skin rash and inflammation of air passages and conjuctival membranes.

Menses: (Latin = months) – discharge of blood and tissue debris at monthly 'period'.

Mentals: symptoms relating to the mental state of the person, their mood, ideas and the way they think.

Modality: factors which make symptoms better or worse.

Mucous membranes: surface-linings of body that secrete mucus for example, mouth and guts.

Mumps: acute infection of parotid salivary gland causing swelling of face and neck and occasionally affecting other organs.

Nasal: of the nose.

Nausea: feeling of sickness.

Neuralgia: affection of nerves (often in head and neck) causing intense, intermittent pain.

Nystagmus: continuous involuntary rolling or oscillation of eyeballs.

Occipital: relating to back of the head.

Oedema: abnormal accumulation of fluid in tissues which often 'dents' when depressed with a finger.

Ovaries: egg-producing organ in female pelvis.

Pallor: paleness.

Paresis: partial paralysis or weakness of muscles.

Parotid gland: salivary gland within cheek in front of ear.

Paroxysm: fit of disease of sudden onset and termination.

Particulars: symptoms relating to a part of the person, that can be expressed 'My . . .' (compare with 'Generals').

Patulous: widely spread apart.

Peculiars: strange, rare and peculiar symptoms which relate to the individual and are not common in the illness.

Periosteum: tough membrane covering bones.

Phlegm: thick, shiny mucus produced in respiratory passage.

Photophobia: intolerance of light.

Picture: collection of symptoms which characterise a remedy or a patient with his illness.

Piles: haemorrhoids, anal varicose veins.

Plethoric: appearance indicating excessive supply of blood, usually used in connection with a ruddy complexion.

Pleurisy: inflammation of pleura (membranes covering lungs and lining chest cavity) causing a sharp pain in chest when breathing.

Pneumonia: acute inflammation of lung.

Potency: 'strength' of a remedy.

Prostration: overcome with fatigue or extreme weakness – must lie down.

Ptosis: drooping of eyelids.

Pulse: heart beat felt in an artery.

Pupil: central black circle of eye in centre of iris.

Purulent: containing pus.

Putrid: rotten, suppurating.

Quinsy: abscess behind tonsil.

Rectum: last part of bowel before anus.

Regurgitation: return of stomach contents into mouth.

Respiratory: relating to breathing.

Retching: ineffectual, involuntary efforts to vomit.

Rheumatic pain: pain in joints and muscles, worse in cold and damp.

Rheumatic fever: acute febrile disease with pain and inflammation of joints, which can affect the heart.

Saliva: digestive secretion of salivary glands in mouth.

Scarlet fever: acute infectious disease characterised by fever and a rash of thickly set red spots followed by scaling or flaking skin.

Sciatica: neuralgia of sciatic nerve causing pain down back of thigh and leg.

Secretions: substances produced by cells and discharged for use elsewhere in the body.

Septic: putrefying due to presence of pathogenic (disease-producing) bacteria.

Shingles: an acute disease caused by the chicken pox virus and characterised by extremely sensitive vesicles on an area of skin limited by its nerve supply.

Shock: sudden and disturbing mental or physical impression; also a state of collapse characterised by pale, cold, sweaty skin, rapid, weak, thready pulse, faintness, dizziness and nausea.

Spasms: sudden, violent involuntary muscular contractions.

Sphincter: ring of muscle closing a body orifice.

Sputum: mucus coughed up from chest.

Sternum: breastbone.

Stitch: sudden sharp pain especially in side of body.

Stool: faeces.

Stupor: dazed, drowsy, stupid and helpless state.

Submaxillary gland: salivary gland beneath lower jaw.

Suppurate: fester and secrete pus.

Symptoms: perceived changes in or impaired function of body or mind indicating presence of disease or injury; what the patient complains of.

Tendons: tough fibrous tissue connecting muscles to other parts, usually bones.

Tenesmus: painful and ineffectual urge to pass a stool.

Testicles: male sperm-producing organs lying in scrotum behind penis.

Thrush: *see* Candida

Tonsils: pair of small lymph nodes inside mouth on either side of root of tongue; protects throat but liable to become infected themselves.

Topically: local application of cream, ointment, tincture or other medicine.

Trachea: wind-pipe.

Trauma: physical injury or wound; also unpleasant and disturbing experience causing psychological upset.

Trigeminal nerve: nerve which divides into three and supplies mandibular (jaw), maxillary (cheek) and ophthalmic (eye and forehead) areas.

Ulcer: open sore on internal or external body surface caused by sloughing of necrotic (dead) tissue.

Umbilicus: 'belly button', site of attachment of umbilical cord.

Urethra: the tube down which urine passes from the bladder to outside.

Urticaria: hives; nettlerash; pale or red elevated patches accompanied by severe itching.

Urinary tract: passages and bladder that conduct the urine.

Uvula: soft, conical fleshy mass hanging centrally from soft palate at back of the mouth.

Vertex: top-most part of the head.

Vertigo: dizziness and sensation of rotation.

Vesicles: small round elevated blisters containing clear, watery fluid.

Waterbrash: return of sour, watery liquid into mouth.

Whooping cough: infectious disease characterised by coryza, bronchitis and violent spasmodic cough.

Wry neck: stiff neck causing deformity and contortion; torticollis.

Index